Caring for someone with arthritis

Carers Handbook Series

Caring for someone with arthritis

Jim Pollard

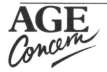

BOOKS

Published by Age Concern England
1268 London Road
London SW16 4ER

First published 2000
Re-issued 2003

Editor Ro Lyon
Production Vinnette Marshall
Designed and typeset by GreenGate Publishing Services, Tonbridge, Kent
Printed in Great Britain by Bell & Bain Ltd, Glasgow

A catalogue record for this book is available from the British Library.

ISBN 0-86242-373-2

The publishers would like to thank Dr Fiona McCrae for her help in updating this book.

Contents

Introduction

This book is aimed at anyone who is or is considering caring for a person with arthritis and wondering whether it is the best way ahead for you both. It gives basic information about arthritis and how it is treated, and raises some of the practical and personal issues you will need to think about if you are to care for somebody with the disease.

Both of you will probably want to read the book, because, as far as possible, it should always be the person being cared for who makes the decisions about their life. That is easily said but hard to do. It's just one of the challenges that caring brings.

I have not been a carer myself but I have seen in my own family the impact that caring and the need for care can have. My personal experience is in working with people with arthritis – for five years I worked for the charity Arthritis Care. I have discussed caring and carers with many disabled people with care needs and it is mainly their views that inform this book. This is not to say that the views of carers are secondary, because I have spoken to many carers too. But when you are considering whether to become a carer, it is important also to bear in mind the views of the person who will be receiving your care.

Whatever you decide, caring is not something that you should drift into – it should be the result of a considered decision. You may find that you have become a carer gradually over time and now want to consider the options that are open to you both. I hope this book will help you make a choice.

Jim Pollard

1 What is arthritis?

This chapter gives a broad overview of the six main categories of arthritis. There then follows more detailed information on the common types, with emphasis on osteoarthritis and rheumatoid arthritis.

Unless you have arthritis, it can sometimes be difficult to understand the problems that the condition can bring, so the chapter includes comments from people saying what it is like for them. Of course, everyone is different, and the person you are caring for will not necessarily agree with all the views expressed, but this helps to emphasise just how important it is to discuss the issues that arthritis raises.

Joy

'I got arthritis in 1972 as the result of a road traffic accident, a car crash. I suffered disc compression in the spine and my walking was affected. However, at first they put my subsequent problems down to stress from the accident.

'I was working as a nurse then on a children's fracture ward, but even so it seemed like the end of the world. It's the not knowing. If you don't know what's happening, you can't come to terms with it and move forward.

'While I was still off sick after the accident, I was sent to a rehabilitation unit where the doctor said there was more wrong than I'd been told. I've a lot to thank him for. He sent me to a rheumatology unit. All in all, it took 18 months before my arthritis was diagnosed.

'A lot of problems are caused by other people's attitudes. I don't want sympathy and I don't want to be patronised ... I could have knocked the block off one rheumatologist! Now I'm better able to talk to doctors but it's only come with experience. I usually know more about arthritis than they do.'

From *Getting a Grip: Self-help for Arthritis and Rheumatism* by Jim Pollard (Headline 1996)

What arthritis is

Two myths about arthritis

One of the great myths about arthritis is that it affects only older people. In fact, according to Arthritis Care and the Arthritis Resarch Campaign, arthritis is the major cause of physical disability in the UK, affecting nine million people – including about 12,000 children.

The second great myth about arthritis is that it is trivial. Because it is so widespread, because nobody will die from arthritis alone and because everyone knows someone who has it, even if it's only the family pet, people assume that it is not serious. Unless you yourself have the disease, it is often very hard to appreciate just how difficult it can be and in how many ways.

The media tend to present two contrasting images of arthritis. The first reinforces the view that it is something trivial that happens only to older people. The second, arising out of the media's general stereotype of disabled people, is rather the opposite: that it is something terrible that leaves you in a wheelchair and dependent.

These images are confusing. And inaccurate. Arthritis is rarely trivial, but using a wheelchair does not mean giving up your independence.

Professionals in the health and social services, who should know better, can be as guilty of falling for these myths as the rest of us. When you care for someone with arthritis, you have the additional challenges of trying to get the disease taken seriously and, in some cases, getting it believed at all.

An overview of arthritis

The name 'arthritis' comes from the Greek *arthron* meaning 'joint' and *itis* meaning 'inflammation'. There are as many as 100 different types of the disease, and it is a feature of about 100 other diseases. Some types of arthritis do not feature inflammation but all involve the joints. You will hear different terms used. Some doctors talk of rheumatic or musculo-skeletal disorders; some patients talk about their rheumatism. They are all talking about what this book calls arthritis. The disease is caused by a number of factors but exactly how and why are still far from fully understood by medical science. Nevertheless, you don't need detailed knowledge about the condition to care for someone with arthritis.

The one thing that can be said with certainty is that arthritis is different for everyone who has it. It is always important to listen to the patient, whatever the disease, but in arthritis it is more important than most. The information in this book is for guidance only. Don't be surprised if the person you are caring for doesn't fit neatly into any of the categories discussed here.

There are six broad categories of arthritis:

- **Osteoarthritis** – disease in which the cartilage at the joint wears away, leaving bone rubbing against bone.
- **Inflammatory** – diseases that begin with swelling in the synovial membrane (the inner lining of the capsule around a movable joint and the tendon sheaths), which contains synovial fluid that lubricates a joint or moving tendon. For example, rheumatoid arthritis.

3

- **Periarticular** – diseases that occur outside the joint, where the tendons and ligaments join the bone. For example, ankylosing spondylitis.
- **Crystal** – diseases that result from crystals forming in the joint. For example, gout.
- **Infective** – diseases arising from viruses or bacteria in the joint (or, sometimes, the gut), called reactive arthritis. For example, Reiter's disease.
- **Muscular** – diseases of the muscle. Although not strictly speaking forms of arthritis, the symptoms and the experiences of people with these conditions can be similar. For example, fibrositis, polymyalgia rheumatica (PMR) and fibromyalgia.

Osteoarthritis

Osteoarthritis is the most common form of arthritis. According to the Arthritis Research Campaign, the number of people with osteoarthritis has risen in the past decade, with two million people now visiting their doctor for treatment each year. After heart disease it is the single major cause of disability in adults.

There is a close relationship between age and osteoarthritis: it usually starts in the late 40s, 50s or 60s and is uncommon before the age of 40. Most people over 65 have one or more joints with moderate to severe osteoarthritis: it becomes more common as we age, especially if we do not look after our joints through appropriate use and exercise. Nevertheless, the disease is not simply the inevitable result of ageing, and can affect anyone of any age at any time.

Generally, osteoarthritis develops slowly. The cartilage becomes worn and bony lumps form, which can make the joint look knobbly. Later the bones begin to rub together. This stage can be very painful and cause the joint to change shape.

Osteoarthritis most commonly affects the knees, hips, hands, feet and spine. Because of its many, often tiny, joints – there are over 150 – the spine is particularly vulnerable, with the neck (the cervical region) and the lower back (the lumbar region) most usually affected.

The hips are more usually affected in men, the knees in women – which may say something about the traditional working roles of the sexes. Because of the use to which these joints are subjected, osteoarthritis in the hip and knee may well worsen more quickly than in other joints, some of which can remain relatively unchanged for years.

Although the synovial membrane may become inflamed in some cases, the term osteoarthritis is not particularly accurate because inflammation is not generally involved. Unlike some other types of arthritis, osteoarthritis is not usually a systemic disease (affecting the whole body), it is joint specific. Sites of old sports injuries, for example, are particularly vulnerable. The typical causes of neck pain are good examples of the two ways osteoarthritis problems develop. They may arise from a particular incident – a whiplash injury, for example, in a car accident – or they may develop over a longer period – the result of an awkward sleeping position, poor posture or working position or a combination of all these and more.

Osteoarthritis varies considerably from person to person. Some people with the early stages of osteoarthritis may never realise they have it, whereas others find it very disabling and may eventually need surgery. Because so many people are affected with joint pains, it can be difficult to get osteoarthritis taken seriously even by those who should know better. At its most severe, osteoarthritis is a very painful and disabling condition.

It is important to get osteoarthritis properly diagnosed. Don't be fobbed off with vague talk about 'a natural sign of ageing' or 'the symptoms are difficult to observe clinically'. You need to know if it is osteoarthritis because it will be crucial to get the right balance between rest and exercise. Joints affected by osteoarthritis tend to be more painful at the end of the day and after exercise. On the other hand, they will become stiff if left inactive. Getting the balance right can make the difference between being in control of the disease and being controlled by it.

Rheumatoid arthritis

Rheumatoid arthritis, the most common type of inflammatory arthritis, is more prevalent than one might imagine. This is because, as with osteoarthritis, it can go unnoticed in its early stages. According to Arthritis Care and the Arthritis Research Campaign, about 387,000 people in the UK have rheumatoid arthritis and there are around 12,000 new cases each year.

These facts are important because, although there is some evidence that the incidence and severity of rheumatoid arthritis are decreasing, the longer life expectancy of people in general and of people with rheumatoid arthritis in particular means that there will be more older people with rheumatoid arthritis in the years to come. Today's older people with long-term disabilities brought on by rheumatoid arthritis are among the first. This is another reason to listen to what they say about their experiences.

Rheumatoid arthritis usually begins in the hands and feet. It generally comes on in relatively early life – before the age of 40 – but people in their 70s and 80s may also develop the condition. It affects three times as many women as men.

The disease occurs as the body's immune system malfunctions. Instead of protecting the body as it should, the immune system turns on it and attacks it. Inflammation, which is a good thing when the auto-immune system is working properly (a sign that the body is successfully repelling invaders), becomes an enemy within. These attacks can be severe – the immune system tends to shoot first and ask questions later. Inflammation of the synovial membrane around the joint causes damage to the ligaments, tendons, cartilage and the joint itself.

It is not only the joints that are affected in rheumatoid arthritis, it is the whole body. Debilitating tiredness and aching muscles, similar to a severe bout of flu, are very common. The eyes, skin and, in a few cases, other organs, may also be affected. For this reason, rheumatoid arthritis is often referred to as rheumatoid disease. Blood tests are commonly used to aid diagnosis.

The disease may appear suddenly – this is more common in older people – or it may come on slowly – the more likely pattern in younger people. It gradually affects more joints over a period of months or it may be what doctors call 'palindromic', flaring up and easing again intermittently before finally setting in. These flare-ups, or flares, are also common in active rheumatoid arthritis.

In contrast with osteoarthritis, rheumatoid arthritis tends to affect the joints in a symmetrical way – both hands, both hips, both knees or both feet. Joint stiffness is more likely in the morning than in the evening.

In about one-third of cases of rheumatoid arthritis, the disease is fairly mild and does not cause severe long-term problems. Another third of patients will be moderately affected, and a further third will have what doctors term more 'aggressive' disease. At the point of diagnosis, it can be difficult to be certain into which category an individual will fall. However, doctors should try to assess this, because there is evidence that early and perhaps heavy drug intervention can reduce the likelihood of more severe disability later. What is more, most joint damage from rheumatoid arthritis occurs in the first two or three years, so early treatment is vital.

One way of estimating the likely development of the disease is through a blood test. Although it is not found in everybody with rheumatoid arthritis, there is some evidence that people with a particular protein in their blood – called rheumatoid factor – may go on to develop more severe rheumatic disease. (For more about rheumatoid factor, see page 24.)

Today's researchers are very interested in the way the immune system works and the way the body deals with inflammation. However, the immune system is an incredibly complex one and researchers stress that it will be a long time before they know whether their current approaches will be successful. You should take any medical breakthrough story you hear about in the media with a pinch of salt. In the case of arthritis, make it an especially large pinch!

Other types of arthritis

Ankylosing spondylitis

This may be the most difficult to pronounce of all the forms of arthritis but is actually very appropriately named. *Ankylosing* is from the Greek for 'stiffness' while *spondylitis* means 'inflammation of the spine'. After osteoarthritis and rheumatoid arthritis, ankylosing spondylitis is the third most common rheumatic disorder in the UK – affecting about 200,000 people, according to the Arthritis Research Campaign.

The disease affects more men than women – the ratio may be as high as five to one – and the usual age of onset is the late teens or early twenties. It usually starts in the lower back, the inflammation going on to cause the formation of bony scar tissue between the vertebrae. Untreated, this tissue will eventually fill the space between the bones and become bone itself, causing the joint to become rigid. This locking of the spine can be prevented by prompt diagnosis and treatment (the usual treatment is exercise). Over the years, the pain and stiffness tend to come and go, often disappearing completely by the age of 55 or 60.

Gout

Because its cause is precisely known, an attack of gout can be readily cured.

For most of us the uric acid in our blood is passed in our urine. Sometimes, however, for reasons that are not fully understood, crystals of uric acid can grow in the cartilage or joint space and the inflammation that results causes the swelling of gout. It usually affects the feet, especially the big toe, the ankles, hands and wrists. An attack, although lasting only a few days, can be very painful and may damage the cartilage.

Drugs and diet can reduce the amount of uric acid in the body. Losing weight may also help. If anti-inflammatory drugs are used, aspirin should be avoided because it can increase the level of uric acid.

Contrary to popular belief, gout is not caused by excess food or drink. However, certain types of either (those which are rich in purines) can make matters worse:

- **Food:** game; pâté; offal (liver, sweetbreads and kidney); some fish (shellfish, fish roe, salmon, herring and whitebait); yeast and its extracts; strawberries; rhubarb; spinach; and asparagus.
- **Drink:** port; and carbonated drinks, including beer, champagne and sparkling wine.

Lupus

Although it is treatable by rheumatologists, systemic lupus erythematosus (usually called 'SLE' or simply 'lupus') is not, strictly speaking, a type of arthritis. Rather, arthritis is a symptom of lupus, which is a disease of the auto-immune system. There is joint and muscle pain, fever and flu-like symptoms. Like rheumatoid arthritis, lupus can be mild or severe, and an up-and-down affair over the years, flaring up and then easing off. Sunlight (or even ultraviolet light from fluorescent lights) can sometimes trigger a flare-up in affected people.

Lupus is rare but seems to be increasing. The number of people with SLE in the UK is estimated to be about 10,000. Doctors are getting better at detecting the disease and this alone may explain the increase. They are also getting better at treating it, with the result that, although lupus remains a serious systemic disease, it is seldom fatal.

It affects far more women than men – the ratio is eight or nine to one – and is most common among women of child-bearing age.

Although the joints are painful, they are rarely damaged. The tendons, the skin and, in some cases, other organs of the body may become inflamed, particularly the kidneys. This inflammation can cause pains that may not at first seem obviously related to lupus. For example, chest pains may be the result of inflammation in the lungs.

Reactive arthritis

Arthritis can occur as a result of an infection, although it may not be immediately obvious that this is what has happened. Six weeks or so may elapse between the infection appearing and the subsequent joint inflammation. It is important to appreciate that, even after the infection has cleared up, arthritis may still remain or, indeed, appear for the first time. This type of arthritis is much more common in men than in women.

The arthritis does not generally last very long, usually going into remission after a few months. A characteristic is that it moves around from one joint to another. Larger joints are most commonly affected – the knee, elbow or ankle are typical – and it rarely hits both of a pair of joints. Sometimes tendons become inflamed.

Two main types of infection can lead to reactive arthritis. One is the infection of the bowel with *Salmonella* or a similar germ – the type that usually results in food poisoning. The second is a sexually transmitted infection. Most sexually transmitted diseases (STDs) can cause arthritis. The commonest is the 'non-specific urethritis' caused by the *Chlamydia* organism. Arthritis may also appear as a complication of an infection elsewhere in the body, such as chickenpox or mumps.

In reactive arthritis, inflammation occurs in the synovial membrane around the joints and may be more painful in the morning. Reiter's disease is a type of reactive arthritis in which inflammation also occurs in the eye (resulting in conjunctivitis or iritis).

Psoriatic arthritis (psoriatic arthropathy)

The skin disease *psoriasis* – from the Greek word for 'itch' – is fairly common, usually affecting the elbows, knees and scalp. The skin becomes inflamed and red, and can seem scaly. It is not contagious and has nothing to do with an individual's personal hygiene.

A skin cell usually lives for a month or so, working its way to the skin's surface where it simply flakes off. Psoriatic cells pack all their activity into a week, dragging live cells with them to the skin's surface and causing a rash.

Psoriatic arthritis is not, strictly speaking, a single disease. Psoriasis accompanies a number of types of arthritis. It can appear, seemingly by coincidence, in rheumatoid arthritis. It can also appear with ankylosing spondylitis. Or it may signify another type of arthritis entirely. The exact connection is unclear but all conditions feature inflammation and a tendency to wax and wane over time.

Sjögren's syndrome

This is another type of auto-immune condition, and affects mostly middle-aged and post-menopausal women. It has also been shown to be occasionally linked to hepatitis C infection. In Sjögren's syndrome the immune system prevents the exocrine glands (eg the saliva and sweat glands) from properly secreting their substances. It results in dry eyes and dry mouth, and is usually accompanied by inflammatory arthritis – such as rheumatoid arthritis or lupus.

Other symptoms are similar to those in other auto-immune diseases: flu-like symptoms and skin rashes. The kidneys and liver may become involved in a few cases. The arthritis is treated in the same way as other systemic (ie not joint-specific) forms, while artificial tears and saliva are employed to do what the glands cannot.

Muscular rheumatic conditions

Some doctors are often sceptical about conditions in which the pain seems to be caused in the muscles rather than the joints. It is very difficult to detect this sort of pain clinically – it won't show up on X-rays – so some doctors might claim that it is 'all in the mind'. And, because the joints aren't directly involved, some rheumatologists don't think this sort of thing is their province anyway. They might try to refer a patient to a neurologist or psychiatrist. None of this is good news for the people who have these conditions.

Look up 'fibrositis' or 'polymyalgia rheumatica' (PMR) in a medical dictionary and, if you find anything at all, you will probably see them described as rare. People working in the arthritis field are less convinced.

Fibrositis

Fibrositis, which is caused by the muscles never really relaxing, is probably quite common among people over 50. Constant muscular tension puts strain on the ligaments, causing pain and disturbing sleep. Relaxing the muscles through appropriate exercise, which may also improve posture, can help. So can relaxation techniques.

Polymyalgia rheumatica (PMR)

As far as symptoms are concerned, polymyalgia rheumatica has much in common with inflammatory arthritis. It is often accompanied by flu-like illness and fatigue, and stiffness is more pronounced in the morning. The disease itself actually affects the muscles. It is rare in people under 50, but is probably more common than often thought in people over this age.

The muscular pain is noticeably different from that experienced after over-exertion or exercise. The inflammation may involve the blood vessels over the skull, resulting in tender temples and perhaps some pain on chewing (called temporal arteritis). Polymyalgia rheumatica will also affect a person's erythrocyte sedimentation rate (ESR), which can be measured by a simple blood test (for more about ESR, see page 24). Certainly, if polymyalgia rheumatica is suspected and the doctor does not offer a blood test, one should be requested.

The condition responds quickly and well to steroid treatment, although it may last for a year or two.

Fibromyalgia

Fibromyalgia is another condition for which no explanation has been found. As well as muscular aches and pains, sleep patterns are disturbed and people feel fatigued. Tender spots around the body are common, but blood tests and x-rays are all normal. A programme of graduated exercises and a low dose of amitriptyline (an antidepressant) have been shown to be of value.

Osteoporosis

Osteoporosis is a bone disease rather than a joint disease but is often found in people with arthritis, particularly older people. Bone cells are constantly being replaced, like those in any organ. The process slows with ageing (bone is strongest at between 30 and 40 years of age) and can, if it slows too much, cause the bony tissue to be replaced with fatty tissue and the bones to become thinner and more brittle and fracture more easily – osteoporosis. This is the most common cause of hip fracture. It is more common in fair-skinned people and among those who are lightly built.

According to the National Osteoporosis Society, 1 in 3 women and 1 in 12 men in the UK will have osteoporosis over the age of 50 – an estimated 3 million people suffer from the disease and every 3 minutes someone has a fracture due to osteoporosis.

Osteoporosis tends to run in families. If your mother has broken her hip, then you are much more likely to break yours too. The risk of the disease is also increased by:

- lack of exercise;
- early menopause (under 45 years old);
- the use of oral steroids – which are used in treating arthritis – over a sustained period;
- low intake of calcium and vitamin D, particularly in childhood; and
- certain other diseases such as those of the liver, thyroid or lungs.

These risks are increased by smoking cigarettes and drinking too much alcohol.

In osteoarthritis the bone mass tends to increase, so people with this type of arthritis may be at less risk of osteoporosis. Having said that, this effect may well be offset by the side (unwanted) effects of typical arthritis drugs, as mentioned above. This is certainly the case in rheumatoid arthritis. Here the risk of osteoporosis is also higher because oral steroids can deplete the bones' calcium.

The menopause is an important watershed because the female hormone oestrogen stimulates the production of vitamin D and calcitonin, which help maintain bone mass. Not surprisingly, the risk of osteoporosis increases when production of this hormone stops. Reduced height after the menopause may be an indication of bone weakness.

For post-menopausal women at risk of osteoporosis, hormone replacement therapy (HRT) used to be an option. HRT involves taking oestrogen by mouth, through a skin patch or gel or by means of a small implant beneath the skin. However, as evidence now suggests that HRT increases the risk of heart disease and stroke, many doctors have changed their recommendations to using HRT for menopausal symptoms only; no longer for the treatment or prevention of osteoporosis in older women. Selective estrogen receptor modulating drugs (SERMs) have recently been developed to have HRT effects only on bone – they appear to protect against breast cancer and not to increase the risk of heart disease or stroke. The only SERM currently licensed for osteoporosis is called Raloxifene.

Bisphosphonate treatments, such as Alendronate and Risedronate, are also now used for osteoporosis in post-menopausal women and men over 45. They can be taken as injections for people in severe osteoporotic pain or who cannot take them orally. Another new treatment is a parathyroid hormone analogue, which works to treat osteoporosis in a different way, and may be useful in patients who need an alternative to bisphosphonates. There is also increasing access to special scans to detect osteoporosis (called dual energy X-ray acquisition scans or DEXA).

Some specific exercises can help once the bone mass is reduced but osteoporosis is best prevented at an earlier stage by a healthy diet, particularly in childhood, and through regular weight-bearing exercise, especially in middle age and upwards. Weight-bearing exercise means just that. Swimming, for example, while a great form of exercise is not weight-bearing. Walking is. Exercise is discussed in more detail on pages 38–44.

Because prevention is better than cure, younger people with arthritis, particularly younger women with rheumatoid arthritis, need to be aware of the long-term risks of osteoporosis.

The main problems caused by arthritis

This section gives an overview of some of the types of problems that can be caused by arthritis. Obviously the detail will vary from individual to individual.

The information here needs to be seen in context. Yes, arthritis is serious. Yes, the problems it brings can be major ones. But no, it is not the end of the world. It might just seem like it as you read the next few paragraphs. That's OK. That's how most people with arthritis feel when they are first diagnosed. But, as the rest of this book will demonstrate, the majority of the difficulties can be overcome. Most people with arthritis can lead the lives they want. Some even say that arthritis is one of the best things that ever happened to them because it has taught them so much about themselves.

Pain

For most people with arthritis, the main symptom is pain. An Arthritis Research Campaign survey in 2002 found that 50 per cent of people with arthritis said that pain was the worst aspect (rising to 55 per cent of people with osteoarthritis). Sometimes the pain is very severe; often it is continual.

As we all know, the physical sensation of pain is bad enough but that is not all it brings. Pain can make it difficult to do everyday things – even turning the pages of this book. It can make movement difficult both for the person with arthritis and for any carer trying to help them to move. To be lifted, even touched, can be excruciating. Pain is mentally as well as physically draining: it can make you tired and erode your self-confidence. Unchecked pain can send anyone into a downward spiral. (For more about pain control in relation to arthritis see pages 49–52.)

The experience of pain and the ability to cope with it vary from individual to individual. The only person who really knows how bad the pain is is the person feeling it. It is an area where you simply cannot make judgements based on your own experience, even your own experience of arthritis.

Lack of mobility

Both damaged joints and painful joints can be difficult to move. People with arthritis in the lower body, including the hips and knees, may well have difficulty with walking and sitting. Some may use a wheelchair. People with the disease in the upper body, particularly the hands and fingers, will have problems with many of the ordinary tasks of day-to-day living. Nearly all of these will be the sort of thing most of us take for granted, so you need to think hard about what the person you are caring for may have trouble with. Undoing a jar, turning a key, switching on an appliance, turning a tap on or off – the list is longer than you think. The little things add up, so it can become difficult to wash or dress oneself. Outside, even if it is possible to get down the steps from the house, is it feasible to get to the nearest shop?

Fatigue

Dealing on a daily basis with pain and lack of mobility can be exhausting. With inflammatory types of arthritis, the disease itself can also be very tiring. There may be flu-like and feverish symptoms, which can be very severe. Imagine the worst flu you've ever had and then some. Many people with arthritis will joke that it affects the brain. It doesn't, of course, but pain and tiredness do have an impact on memory and concentration.

What arthritis will *not* affect is anyone's capacity to make decisions. In fact, it can be argued that disability is good for the brain because disabled people become experts at detailed thinking and coming up with solutions to problems.

What is disability?

More people are disabled by arthritis than by any other medical condition. But what images spring to mind when you think about disabled people?

There are usually two main ones – victim or hero. The media particularly like the heroes – people who have triumphed over their disability and achieved despite it. Examples involving people with arthritis include the woman who climbed Everest, the boy who got a degree, the girl who does ballet and the man who ran a marathon. They think these stories sell newspapers. Most are patronising, and they all dwell on the strangeness of difference. Meanwhile, the charities often emphasise the victim image in order, they believe, to obtain people's sympathy and donations.

It's no wonder that the general public are so scared of X disease or Y impairment. They know they are not heroes so they are terrified of becoming victims. Of course, most people with disabilities aren't heroes or victims at all; they are just ordinary people who happen to have X or Y.

The problem is that these images put a barrier between people with a disability and people without. Think about disability for a moment. Most people, including most doctors, see disability as a medical problem. Disabled people have a disease that needs to be cured. But *is* the disease the real issue? Imagine the following scenario. You want to go to the cinema but you can't because the cinema has steps outside, which you cannot get up because of the arthritis in your knees. What is really stopping you getting into the cinema – the arthritis or the steps? It is a lot easier, quicker and cheaper to build a ramp than to find a cure for arthritis. Looked at this way, disability becomes a social problem. It is society that disables through the barriers – real and metaphorical – that it places in the way of disabled people. Remove the barriers – whether they are a flight of stairs or individuals' prejudices – and you remove the disability. This is sometimes referred to as the social model of disability. It is a really useful way to begin to see beyond the problems to the solutions.

Of course, it is important to think carefully about the medical aspects of arthritis and to explore any new treatments or ideas but don't become obsessed with finding a cure. Even when cures for arthritis emerge – and it won't be in our lifetimes – they will not help the vast majority of people who have the disease today and certainly not those whose disease is so advanced that they have care needs.

Society, in contrast to damaged joints, can change and is changing. The *Disability Discrimination Act 1995* makes it illegal to discriminate against disabled people in employment, in providing goods and services, and in selling or letting land or property. However, the Act – and this is why it is far from perfect – does allow discrimination if the provider has a justifiable reason for giving less favourable treatment. The Government has set up the Disability Rights Commission to help disabled people secure their rights under the Act and to advise about any 'appropriate subsequent law'. As a carer you can really help disabled people by joining their push towards equality.

What is it like to have arthritis?

Meet two people with arthritis who have different degrees of care needs: Joy and Sarah.

Joy's story

There is no typical arthritis story but Joy's raises many of the issues that people with arthritis consider important. She is in her fifties and has osteoarthritis, the most common form of the disease.

Joy

'After arthritis was diagnosed, I was put on the anti-inflammatory drug ibuprofen and I was on it for 15 years. Eventually I said to my doctor that I was worried my stomach would go. She said, "If your stomach was going to go, it would have gone years ago." Then I got a peptic ulcer. I went back to the doctor and challenged her. She said, "What was the point of my alarming you?"

'I know now that ulcers are a not uncommon side effect of anti-inflammatory drugs, but if anything the ulcer has been worse in some ways than the arthritis. It was the ulcer that caused my retirement from work.

'When I first had arthritis, it was difficult for everybody I know. People wanted to do too much. Now family and friends know there isn't anything I can't do – it just takes time. Initially, I was terribly ungracious but the truth is: if you don't know how to handle your arthritis, how can you expect other people to know how to handle it?

'I have been very proud over the years. I didn't want to seem different. Now it doesn't bother me. Sometimes I used a wheelchair at work. It made me self-sufficient. Without it, I couldn't have done half of what I did; I wouldn't have been able to carry anything. Also, I still had enough energy left when I got home to do my housework and voluntary work. But work colleagues found it hard to come to terms with. They would see me walking one day and using a wheelchair the next. They thought I should always be the same or else I was exaggerating on the bad days. They didn't understand that that's how arthritis is. I've stopped trying to justify using the wheelchair some times and not others. If people can't accept me as I am, forget it.

'Arthritis has made me a much better person. I can now appreciate other people's problems much more. Before I had arthritis I used to think that I was sympathetic and understanding, but I didn't really understand; I had no idea. I'm sorry I had to have it but it has enhanced my life – I have much more empathy.'

From *Getting a Grip: Self-help for Arthritis and Rheumatism* by Jim Pollard (Headline 1996)

Sarah's story

Many people with arthritis are carers too. Sarah has arthritis and her husband Peter has a heart condition.

Sarah

'I have osteoarthritis but my husband has had a number of heart attacks so we care for each other. He helps me dress and we try to do the housework between us. But he's one of these blokes who has to do it all at once. He can't do a little at a time. That worries me. He can move around more than me but, because his heart is involved, his condition is potentially more life-threatening.

'I'd like a home help but it would be difficult. My husband wouldn't let me have one when it was first offered after my knee operation. Even now I don't think he'd like it. I think he does more than he should and that makes me feel guilty, as I think I should be doing more. I did much more after his last heart attack but I really paid for it. What's more, people see me walking around and don't realise the problems I have. For example, we have a disabled parking space but the neighbours keep using it. They see me walking and so they resent my having a special space.

'They don't know all the problems I had with my operation. I had to have it done twice. Now the surgeons would like to operate on my spine but I don't want them to. I go to a pain clinic because I've been on painkillers so long I'm beginning to have problems with my stomach. I found a TNS machine that could help but then I developed an allergic reaction to the pads.

'Hydrotherapy helps. The other thing that helps is reducing stress. I felt much better when we went on holiday. But avoiding stress is very hard. As well as Peter's heart, we've had a few problems with our children which hasn't helped the arthritis – it's definitely worse when I feel stressed. I can get depressed, too. With hindsight I think a lot of the bouts of depression that I've had can be put down to arthritis and vice versa. I often wonder exactly how the two are related.

'But there is one advantage in us both having problems. I think it helps us to understand each other's difficulties more.'

For more *i*nformation

i Arthritis Care free booklets (address on page 141):

Information for People with Arthritis

Rheumatoid Arthritis: A Guide

Talk About Pain.

2 How is arthritis treated?

This chapter outlines the main tests that may be carried out to diagnose arthritis. It then looks at the sorts of things a person with arthritis needs to think about when managing their disease. The information will be useful to any carer who wants to understand more about how the disease is treated. It includes treatments that doctors will suggest, such as drugs, but many you will need to seek out for yourself, such as complementary therapies and self-help groups. It should give you a good idea of the sort of people someone with arthritis might want to talk to.

Mei-Lee

'I went to see my GP because, although not exactly in pain, I was very aware of my knees. She tested the movement in my legs and said she could hear a grating sound at my knees, so it might well be osteoarthritis. She sent me to the local hospital for X-rays, and they confirmed her diagnosis.'

Diagnosing arthritis

Osteoarthritis is usually diagnosed readily without X-rays or blood tests. However, if the symptoms are complex, pretty soon the GP should do some blood tests and arrange for an X-ray. Tests are used in four ways:

- to assist in diagnosis;
- to assess the severity of a disease;
- to assess the effects of a treatment; or
- to check for side effects.

Which tests are appropriate will depend on the individual and the type of arthritis. In many larger practices these may be done on the premises by a practice nurse; smaller ones will refer the person to the local hospital.

X-rays will be taken of the painful joints, and possibly also of adjacent joints and of the feet if rheumatoid arthritis is suspected. The feet are X-rayed because the physical changes caused by rheumatoid arthritis often appear there first. Other diagnostic techniques include ultrasound scanning, magnetic resonance imaging (MRI) and bone densitometry (bone density) scans. All these enable the doctor to get an idea of the appearance and state of the bones and joints. They won't show pain – patients need to tell doctors about this themselves.

Blood tests

The study of the blood is called haematology, and blood tests are done in the haematology department. The tests typically used in arthritis are as follows:

Red cell count Red cells contain haemoglobin, which carries oxygen into and carbon dioxide out of the body via the lungs. A low haemoglobin level (anaemia) may indicate a deficiency in iron or vitamins or, in rheumatoid arthritis, disease activity. In this last case, monitoring haemoglobin levels helps monitor the disease: worsening anaemia may suggest a complication. People taking the more powerful anti-arthritis drugs are regularly screened because on rare occasions these drugs may reduce the bone marrow cells that form blood.

The erythrocyte sedimentation rate (ESR) test This test measures the speed at which red blood cells settle under gravity. Inflammation increases the rate of settlement: the quicker the rate, the higher the ESR. A high ESR may, alongside other factors, show that the patient's arthritis is becoming more active and causing more inflammation. On the other hand, it might indicate that there is some other inflammation, and the doctors will have to use their judgement as well as the test results.

The CRP test This monitors levels of the C-reactive protein (CRP) in the blood. As with the ESR, a high level suggests more inflammation due to arthritis. It is rather more specific than the ESR.

White cell count White cells help defend the body against foreign invaders. A rise in their numbers indicates an infection or perhaps, because of the increased auto-immune activity involved, conditions such as rheumatoid arthritis or lupus. The doctor can learn more from closer examination of the three types of white cells (polymorphs, macrophages and lymphocytes) – a rise in one, perhaps, and not the others. A reduced lymphocyte count, for example, is typical of lupus. Drugs can also reduce the number of white cells and this is why patients taking certain stronger drugs need to have a monthly blood test.

Platelet count Platelets are essential for blood-clotting. They are measured because, like white cells, they can be reduced by certain drugs.

Rheumatoid factor At least 70 per cent of people with rheumatoid arthritis have an unusual protein – called rheumatoid factor – in their blood. (People with rheumatoid factor are sometimes termed sero-positive.) It is not the cause of the disease, and many people with the rheumatoid factor never get rheumatoid arthritis. On the other hand, people who get rheumatoid arthritis often develop the rheumatoid factor over time. There is some evidence that people with a particularly high rheumatoid factor develop a more severe disease. The mystery is: why do over three-quarters of people with rheumatoid factor *not* have the condition?

Patient power

You might think that 'patient power' is just another slogan, but it really does work and at absolutely no cost to anyone. Being in control of the management of their arthritis can make people feel better.

David

'One thing I've learned is that there is no one treatment for arthritis. It's not just about taking the drugs – you need to do several things and get a balance between, say, rest and exercise or keeping busy and being relaxed. Nobody will tell you what is best for you; you need to find out for yourself. Make sure your doctors know about the things you're trying, obviously, but don't expect them to know all the answers.'

Well worth considering by anyone with arthritis are courses in self-management and in personal development. Arthritis Care run some excellent ones. These give people with arthritis the opportunity to get together with others with the disease and with trainers who also have arthritis, to share experiences, learn from each other and boost self-esteem.

Anyone who is unsure about such a course is in good company. 'I didn't fancy it all,' says Jean Thompson who has rheumatoid arthritis. 'For thirty years I'd deliberately not had contact with anyone else with arthritis.'

Jean

'I was very sceptical at the start of my course but after three weeks I realised that bringing together people who had nothing in common on the surface other than their arthritis could really work. I learned so much. I realised that my pattern of operating had been damaging my health. I used to have a flare every three years but now I've gone six years without one through listening more to my body. When it's a bad day I don't take anything on. 'Challenging Arthritis' cemented this in me. I began a calmer life. People are empowered by the programme to look after themselves. They meet as equals. The ethos is sharing. Everybody has the opportunity to stand back and reflect. Everybody has the opportunity to be success-ful. I used to do a lot of negative thinking – not now.'

People are equally enthusiastic about personal development courses.

Joyce

'I'm a lot more positive now. I'd recommend a personal development course to anyone. You've got nothing to lose and everything to gain. You just need to be prepared to take a hard look at yourself, which can be dif-ficult.'

The training programmes enable people with arthritis to manage their condition more effectively, often dramatically improving their quality of life.

For more *i*nformation

i For information about courses in self-management and personal develop-ment in your locality, contact Arthritis Care at the address on page 141.

Drug treatments

A key way of controlling arthritis is by medication. Most people with the condition will be taking prescribed drugs (medicines), often more than one and often over a prolonged period. It is important that the person with the disease knows what they are taking and why. As a carer you can help them to do this – by mak-ing sure the doctor explains everything fully, for example – but the organisation and maintenance of their drug regimen is not, in most cases, something that it is helpful for you to take over. However, you can both read the information on the drug packaging. If either of you has any questions, ask the pharmacist to explain. Many pharmacies will now dispense drugs in weekly boxes which lay all the drugs out by time of day and day of the week. All the drugs for each time period are together, so that the person with arthritis can simply take the drugs in the appropriate chamber for the time and day. This has an added advantage of showing the drugs that have been forgotten.

This section includes basic information on the main types of drugs used to treat arthritis. It is not for self-prescription but should enable you and the person you are caring for to quiz the doctor more effectively.

All drugs used in the UK must be licensed by the Medicines Control Agency. It checks that research and trials have been conducted to a sufficient standard and indicates how the product may be used. There are three categories:

- **prescription-only drugs**, which are prescribed by a doctor or dentist and supplied by a pharmacist;
- **pharmacy medicines**, or 'over-the counter' medicines, which can be bought without a prescription but only in a pharmacist/chemist shop (eg stronger painkillers); and
- **general sales list (GSL) drugs**, which can be bought pretty much anywhere, including supermarkets.

The last group includes paracetamol, ibuprofen and aspirin. Buying these drugs by their generic (chemical) names is cheaper than buying them by their more familiar brand names (such as Panadol, Nurofen or Anadin).

All drugs, even those only on the general sales list, can have side effects. Side effects are a fact of life. All drugs, from coffee to cocaine, have them. Many will be pretty harmless but some may be dangerous. Make sure that the person with arthritis knows what these risks are and what to look out for. It is the doctor's responsibility to make sure the patient understands. It is the patient's responsibility to report a possible side effect as soon as possible.

In arthritis treatment, drugs can do three things:

■ relieve pain;
■ reduce inflammation; and
■ help suppress disease activity.

Doing these things can cause side effects, and other drugs may be prescribed to offset them. It is important *always* to follow the instructions given for each drug, and never to exceed the stated dose.

Drug treatments for osteoarthritis

Treatment for osteoarthritis is aimed at controlling pain and stiffness. Most people start with simple painkillers (**analgesics**) and/or creams, gels and rubs, before resorting to anti-inflammatory drugs, because of the risk of side effects (see below) – eight paracetamol in divided doses per day is safer in the long term than one anti-inflammatory tablet per day.

Analgesics

Analgesics reduce pain. Some of these painkillers, such as paracetamol and paracetamol with codeine, can be bought over the counter. Recent legislation prevents the purchase of more than 32 tablets in one go. Other painkillers in increasing strength are: coproxamol, cocodamol, codydramol (these three contain paracetamol); then dihydrocodeine, tramadol, and buprenorphine. These are called **narcotics** and are available on prescription only. Narcotics mimic the action of the body's natural painkillers (called endorphins) and block the transmission of pain within the brain. They contain weak opiate drugs. Extremely potent opiate drugs (derived from morphine and heroin) are available for severe pain, sometimes as patches. The stronger the painkiller the greater the risk of more side effects of constipation and drowsiness and confusion.

Creams, gels and rubs

Creams, gels and rubs – such as ibuprofen cream, Ralgex, Deep Heat, etc – are available over the counter. They can be useful when symptoms are minor or limited to one or two joints, or the person with arthritis doesn't want to take tablets. The risk of these causing unwanted side effects is low, but sometimes they are not very effective.

Capsaicin cream works differently from other creams by overwhelming the pain sensors (the main constituent – chilli – is well known for the same effect on taste). Some people, but not all, get good relief of symptoms, but care must be taken not to get it near sensitive parts such as the eyes or genitals.

Anti-inflammatory drugs

Anti-inflammatory drugs (which are also known as non-steroidal anti-inflammatory drugs or **NSAIDs**) can be used if painkillers in full dose are not sufficient to control symptoms. They help both pain and stiffness. For many people they restore a reasonable quality of life. For these people the benefits outweigh the risk.

It is preferable not to use these drugs for prolonged periods, however, because of their long-term side effects. Conventional NSAIDs, such as ibuprofen, diclofenac, naproxen, indomethacin, and many others, can cause stomach or duodenal ulceration. This can occur without any symptoms. If undetected these ulcers can (very rarely) perforate or bleed. Other side effects of NSAIDs include anaemia, increased blood pressure, kidney impairment, liver impairment, fluid retention and precipitation of an asthma attack.

Newer NSAIDs, called **COX-2 inhibitors**, have been designed to work without the risk to the stomach or duodenum. These are rofecoxib, celecoxib, meloxicam, and etodolac. The National Institute for Clinical Excellence (NICE) has indicated that these drugs should replace the conventional NSAIDs for people over 65, or with a history of peptic ulcer, or heart disease, or on steroids. It may be possible to continue with a preferred conventional NSAID instead, however, if a drug to protect the stomach is used as well. The COX-2 inhibitor drugs carry the same risk of side effects on blood pressure, kidney and liver impairment, and fluid retention as the conventional drugs.

Drug treatments for inflammatory arthritis (rheumatoid arthritis and psoriatic arthritis)

Analgesics and NSAIDs (see above) are considered the first line of treatment in inflammatory arthritis. Anti-inflammatory drugs are used earlier than in osteoarthritis, because the stiffness in inflammatory arthritis is much greater than in osteoarthritis and not relieved by analgesics alone. These drugs do not stop the underlying damage that occurs in inflammatory arthritis, so other additional treatments are recommended as early as possible to reduce the risk of joint damage. No curative treatment is yet available, but the control of the disease has improved greatly in the last few years, mostly because of the increased use of methotrexate, and the use of combinations of drugs.

Other drugs for inflammatory arthritis include sulphasalazine, gold, D penicillamine, azathioprine and hydroxychloroquine. Leflunomide is a newer drug which has been made available recently. All these drugs are slow acting – taking several weeks to start working. First-line drugs such as painkillers and NSAIDs are continued during this time to control symptoms. Once the slow-acting drugs start working, the levels of pain and stiffness reduce and the person with arthritis often feels generally better in themselves. Occasionally, but not always, they are able to discontinue the first-line drugs. Each of these drugs requires careful monitoring because of the risk of side effects described below.

Methotrexate

Methotrexate is currently the 'gold standard' treatment of rheumatoid arthritis. All new drugs are compared to methotrexate. Its brand names include Emtexate and Maxtrex). Common combinations often include methotrexate sulphasalazine, and hydroxychloroquine. It is used in large doses to treat some cancers and also works directly on the cells involved in the immune process, so it is also classed as a 'chemotherapy' drug and 'immunosuppressant'. It is taken once weekly, so is best given on the same day every week. Folic acid is often prescribed to take a day or two later to reduce the incidence of mouth ulcers.

The major side effects of methotrexate are on liver function and reducing the number of blood cells. These effects can be detected by regular blood tests and the drug stopped before the person is aware of any illness. It is important to avoid alcohol, or at least cut consumption right down, when taking methotrexate as this drug will accelerate liver cirrhosis. A rare complication of methotrexate is pneumonitis which starts with sudden breathlessness and cough. If any of these symptoms occur it is important to tell the doctor. Because methotrexate affects the body's immune system it can also impair the ability to fight infection, so treatment with antibiotics may be required more often. Methotrexate has the advantage of being an effective treatment for psoriasis as well as arthritis. Some patients switch to injections of methotrexate if stomach upsets or lack of effect is a problem with the tablet. Live vaccinations (ie those for polio, rubella and yellow fever) should be avoided by people on immunosuppressive drugs such as methotrexate; 'flu and pneumoccal vaccinations are recommended, however.

Sulphasalazine

This drug is nearly as effective as methotrexate. It is not classed as chemotherapy or an immunosuppressant; its mode of action is not clearly understood. Once a person has taken it for a few months it is relatively safe. In the first few weeks of treatment queasiness or bowel upsets are common side effects and for that reason the dose is usually built up slowly. There is also a risk of problems with the blood cells in the first four to six months of treatment, so regular blood tests are required. Rashes are occasionally a problem. The urine turns orange – as do tears which can stain contact lenses orange. In men the sperm count can be reduced, which can cause infertility (but not impotence). Liver function is checked with each blood test, but there is no requirement to avoid alcohol while taking this drug. It is usually prescribed as Salazopyrin EN (coated tablets).

Gold (myocrisin) injections

When gold works it has a dramatically beneficial effect, and the person tends to feel a general sense of well-being. Unfortunately, gold is not always effective and the practical issues surrounding the administration of gold and the relatively high risk of unwanted side effects is making it less popular. It is given by injection (of a solution of gold salts) every week for several months, and then the frequency reduced so that after a while the gold is given only every month or so. The injection cannot be self administered, so the person may have to attend their local surgery or hospital, unless arrangements are made for a nurse to visit. Each injection has to be preceded by a blood test and a urine test.

Side effects which can be caused by gold are a reduction in the number of blood cells, and the kidneys leaking protein. Both these side effects can be serious and recovery can take some time. Rashes are also quite common, as well as mouth ulcers. Some people experience a metallic taste in the mouth.

D penicillamine

This is an older drug which is reducing in popularity. Like gold, when it works the effects can be dramatic, but the chance of effectiveness is relatively low and the risk of side effects is relatively high. It is given in a daily tablet form and the dose gradually increased. Its brand name is Distamine. The potential side effects again relate to the blood cells and kidneys, so regular blood and urine tests are required. D penicillamine can also (but only rarely) be responsible for causing other diseases such as lupus, although this is reversible on withdrawal from the drug. A temporary loss of taste can also occur at the beginning of the treatment. It must be taken on an empty stomach.

Azathioprine

This is a well-established drug treatment which is also classed as chemotherapy and as an immunosuppressant. It is used for both inflammatory arthritis and lupus. Brand names include Azamune and Imuran. It is usually easily tolerated, although occasionally rashes can occur, and queasiness in the first few days of treatment. Some people have a peculiar reaction to azathioprine, which shows in the blood as reduced cell counts. For this reason frequent blood tests are required in the first few weeks of treatment, and intermittent tests thereafter.

A new drug called mycophenylate mofetil has similar actions to azathioprine and is gaining popularity in the treatment of lupus.

Leflunomide

This drug was introduced in 1999, and has been shown to be on a par with methotrexate in the treatment of rheumatoid arthritis. If loading doses (ie a bigger dose to build up the blood levels in the body quickly) are used, it starts working more quickly than the other second-line drugs. A few patients cannot tolerate loading doses because of headache or diarrhoea, so some rheumatologists are now avoiding the use of the loading dose, and just start the regular dose from the beginning. As with methotrexate, alcohol should be avoided whilst taking this drug, and blood tests are required to look for problems with the cell counts and liver and kidney functions. Regular checks of blood pressure are required as well. Its brand name is Arava.

Hydroxychloroquine

This is an old-fashioned anti-malarial drug which no longer works as a treatment for malaria, but is recognised as a good treatment for the joint pain and skin rash of lupus, and sometimes very effectively as a treatment for rheumatoid arthritis, often in combination with other drugs. Its brand name is Plaquenil. It is considered pretty safe, and does not require monitoring blood tests. At the start of treatment an itchy skin rash can appear, and has to be treated by stopping the drug. Over many years of treatment there is potential risk of molecules of the drug getting deposited at the back of the eye, which, if not detected, could affect the person's vision. For this reason people taking the drug should be screened by an optician or ophthalmologist about once a year.

TNF blocking drugs

TNF stands for **tumour necrosis factor**, which plays a key role in the inflammation of rheumatoid arthritis. These drugs are also called **biologics** and include infliximab, etanercept and adalimumab. The first two were approved by NICE in 2002. They are probably the most effective treatment currently available for the treatment of rheumatoid arthritis, with almost instant beneficial effect, doing away with the delay in response to the other second-line agents. However, they have been reserved for use in patients with severe rheumatoid arthritis, who have failed to respond to treatment with methotrexate, and whose disease is shown to be very active, as measured by blood tests, a questionnaire and by number of inflamed joints. The reason for this restriction of use is partly due to cost, as these drugs are very much more expensive than methotrexate, but also because of the lack of long-term information about the safety of the treatment. The research studies have so far followed patients for only a few years, and longer-term effects may still be found. Already there is evidence of reactivation of tuberculosis in patients treated with TNF blocking drugs and a suspicion of increased risk of multiple sclerosis in some people. Susceptibility to infection may be increased, and there is some theoretical risk of bone marrow cancers. Treatment is not advised in patients who have had cancer within the last 10 years, as the treatment might reawaken the cancer. The patient will be entered onto a register held by the British Society for Rheumatology which is keen to audit the national use of these drugs.

Infliximab is given by intravenous infusion (usually as a day case in hospital) every eight weeks, and etanercept by twice weekly injection into the tummy or legs (this can be done by the person themselves). No particular blood tests are required, but blood tests will be carried out intermittently to keep an eye on the arthritis itself.

Adalimumab is given by self injection every other week. Anakinra is another biologic drug newly launched for rheumatoid arthritis. It has a different mode of action from TNF blockers, but shows similar potential.

Steroids

Steroids (such as prednisolone, prednisone, medrone, depomedrone, triamcinolone) are used in many ways to help patients with arthritis. Their effect is a rapid and effective reduction of inflammation. Most commonly steroids are given as injections into joints or soft tissues near joints. This method helps the injected joint to settle, without causing any unwanted side effects elsewhere. Injected joints should be rested for 24 to 48 hours. Occasionally the person gets a red face for 24 hours after the injection. The joint might feel worse after the injection for a few hours; usually the pain settles within two days (in rare cases it takes up to a week).

Intramuscular depomedrone (ie injection of steroid into the large muscle of the leg, buttock or arm) is an effective way of switching off a flare of rheumatoid arthritis. It is quite common to be given this injection in the rheumatology clinic on the same day as a second-line drug is started. A single intramuscular steroid injection has few general side effects, but if the injection is given repeatedly the risk of steroid side effects becomes more pronounced.

Intravenous methyl prednisolone 'pulse' treatment gives the patient a higher dose with more rapid effect than intramuscular depomedrone, and is given in severe flares of rheumatoid arthritis, often as part of an admission to hospital or as a day case.

Oral steroids (tablets) are helpful in settling arthritis quickly, and have some long-term benefit in slowing down the rate of damage to the joints. Low doses of prednisolone (brand names include Deltacortril Enteric, Precortisyl, Prednesol and Sintisone) are often used either on their own, or in addition to a second-line agent.

Doctors are a little wary of higher doses and long-term use of steroids because of the side effects. These are:

- weight gain;
- increased facial hair;
- thin, easily bruising skin;
- thin bones (prone to fracture – osteoporosis);
- increased blood pressure;
- increased blood sugar (diabetes);
- cataracts;
- depression;
- stretch marks;

- difficulties with wound healing; and
- muscle weakness.

The risk of these side effects increases with dose and duration of treatment. Someone who is taking steroids for more than three weeks should not stop their treatment suddenly; instead, the dose should be gradually reduced. They should carry a steroid card to inform health professionals in the event of an emergency.

Cyclophosphamide (its brand name is Endoxana) and cyclosporin (brand name Sandimmun) are other potent immunosuppressant drugs occasionally used in inflammatory arthritis.

Drug treatments for ankylosing spondylitis

Hydrotherapy is the most important aspect of treatment of anky-losing spondylitis, with long-term use of NSAIDs also important. There is a little evidence emerging that the new TNF blocking drugs may be helpful in severe cases, but these drugs have not yet been licensed for this use.

Drug treatments for gout

Single attacks of gout usually settle with full doses of anti-inflam-matory treatment. People who cannot use NSAIDs (because of kidney failure for example) may benefit from colchicine (an extract of crocus) or even a short course of steroids. Recurrent attacks of gout may need lifelong treatment with allopurinol. This drug reduces the level of uric acid in the body and gradually reduces the frequency of attacks or size of the tophi (gouty lumps). When starting allopurinol an acute attack can be precipi-tated, so it is usually advised that the person also takes their usual treatment for an acute attack for the first two weeks of treatment.

How to get the best out of drugs

When the doctor prescribes drugs for you or the person you are caring for, make sure you know exactly what they are. It can take time to find the right drug and the right dosage. Knowing exactly what is being taken helps you to assess the effects.

Ask the doctor:

- What is the drug called? (Both the brand name and the generic name.)
- How many tablets should be taken and how often? Before or after eating? At bedtime? What if a dose is missed?
- What does it do? Is it a painkiller (analgesic), an anti-inflammatory, an immunosuppressant?
- What specific benefits should it bring?
- How quickly will it work? (Some drugs work more quickly than others.)
- How strong is it? (In milligrams.)
- What are the possible side effects? Is there anything that can be done to prevent them? What should be done if it seems that the person may be experiencing them?
- Should anything be avoided while taking the drug? Alcohol? Driving? Operating machines?

With certain drugs, such as steroids where it is important that the course of treatment is not interrupted, patients are given an information card which should be carried at all times. With others, such as gold, a record card is provided, to be filled in after every treatment and blood and urine test.

Something that is not always stressed enough in the doctor's surgery is the importance of taking the drugs at the right time and in the right quantity. People use all sorts of methods to remind them: watch alarms, kitchen timers, notes in a diary, good-natured partners and so on. You can even buy a beeping pill box. For best results, drugs should be taken according to the clock and the doctor's instructions, not according to how much pain is felt. Lurching from one extreme to the other makes it harder to assess the effectiveness of the medication and can be very disruptive to everyday life.

It helps the doctor to prescribe the right medication if the patient is blunt about how they feel. Being brave or uncomplaining may lead to the wrong drug or a dose that is too low. Too little of a painkiller is more likely to lead to dependence than too much, because the body notices the difference it makes far more. And no one should ever feel guilty if what is first prescribed doesn't work.

Doctors usually have a system to work through, starting with the most commonly effective drug and dose, and then trying others according to the individual's responses.

Patients should be frank with their doctor about side effects. With NSAIDs, for example, a number of strategies can be employed to reduce stomach pain: spreading the dose (more frequent doses of weaker tablets); changing the time at which the dose is taken (eg after eating when the stomach lining is coated); trying a coated tablet (which will pass through the stomach before releasing its contents); or taking an antacid with the drug. This advice also applies to any over-the-counter aspirin.

Prescriptions can be expensive for most patients between the ages of 18 and 60 and the charge tends to rise every year. Despite lobbying by patients' organisations, a person with arthritis does not qualify for free prescriptions as do some people with other long-term medical conditions (eg diabetes). However, anyone who has to pay for a lot of prescribed drugs may be able to save money by buying a prescription prepayment certificate (PPC). The application form is available from pharmacists or you can order a PPC by ringing 0845 850 00 30.

When buying over-the-counter drugs such as aspirin, ibuprofen or paracetamol, it is cheaper to ask for them by these generic names rather than choose one of the brand names.

For more *i*nformation

i More information about arthritis drugs can be found in Arthritis Care's free booklet *The Balanced Approach: A Guide to Medicines and Complementary Therapies* (address on page 141).

Exercise and leisure activities

The facts about exercise are simple: get enough and you'll feel better, have more energy, be able to do more and might even live longer. People with arthritis need exercise as much as anybody else but must choose more carefully the forms it takes. The fatigue associated with certain types of arthritis and the loss of bone mass in osteoporosis can make a difference to what is appropriate.

Sarah

'We both try to keep active – Peter plays bowls. It's important to keep your mind active as much as anything else. I visit a care home and take some of the residents to church or play the organ. It helps me forget my own problems.'

Leisure activities such as sport and gardening can be continued, even if they may need a bit of modification. For example, Disability Sport England (address on page 144) promotes sport for people with disabilities from local to national level. Sport England (address on page 149) encourages sports governing bodies to cater for older people, and provides information on leadership and the addresses of regional sports councils, which will have more local information. Gardeners with disabilities or special needs can obtain advice and information from Thrive (address on page 150). RADAR (address on page 149) publishes information giving details of accessibility to, for example, places of interest. Some national organisations, such as the National Trust and English Heritage (addresses on pages 148 and 146), publish guides for visitors with disabilities.

People with arthritis enjoy additional benefits from exercising. It protects against joint damage, keeps joints and muscles working, and helps to prevent disability. Unexercised joints can lose muscle strength, becoming painful and unstable, and cartilage deteriorates faster. So rather than resting arthritic joints, it is even more important to exercise them. Someone with osteoarthritis will not do any damage through exercise, even if it causes some pain. Exercise also helps keep bones strong, which can protect against osteoporosis. Moreover, people who are confident on their feet are less likely to have accidents.

Age is no barrier. Studies show that men and women aged 65 and over can improve their strength, stamina and suppleness considerably within a few weeks of beginning a supervised exercise programme. Most forms of exercise can be done with a friend or partner – for example, walking, dancing or taking part in a class – which will make it an enjoyable activity rather than a boring chore.

There are three types of exercise – stretching, strengthening and endurance exercise. A good programme will include all three, and will take into account the type and severity of the arthritis and the individual's general level of fitness. Sports and health centres often have staff who are qualified to give advice, but people with arthritis should probably consult their GP or physiotherapist before beginning any new exercise programme.

Stretching exercise

Stretching or range of movement (ROM) exercise is the most important for people with arthritis. It involves taking your joints through their full range of movement and then just easing them a little further. This is the sort of exercise people do when warming up for sport; it is excellent for maintaining a joint's mobility and over time may well improve it. Stretching exercises can even be performed on inflamed joints.

Joy

'Exercise is vitally important but so is rest. The difficult bit is the balance. Too much rest and you get stiff; too much exercise and you're in pain. I relax in my garden. If I'm uptight I just disappear out there. I don't do much – just a bit of dead-heading or something – but afterwards I'm a different person. I do my stretching exercises anywhere – watching TV, even sitting in the car in traffic jams (I get some funny looks!).'

From *Getting a Grip: Self-help for Arthritis and Rheumatism* by Jim Pollard (Headline 1996)

Strengthening exercise

By tightening and releasing the muscles around a joint, strengthening exercises can help restore its strength and stability. The particular strengthening exercises will depend very much on the location, severity and type of the individual's arthritis. For example, strengthening the quadriceps muscles on the front of the thighs is excellent for arthritis in the knees. Some exercises will be harmful for some people so it is essential to discuss a programme with a health professional. People with painful hips and knees should certainly avoid too many weight-bearing exercises, and heavy weight-lifting is not recommended.

Muscle weakness can be the result of the arthritis itself, of the inactivity it prompts and sometimes of the long-term use of steroid drugs. For this reason some strengthening exercises may be quite difficult at first but they do become easier, especially if done in conjunction with ROM exercise. Strengthening exercise should not be performed on inflamed joints until the pain or swelling has eased, or done only very slowly to minimise the pain.

Endurance exercise

This is the sort of thing we normally think of as exercise – walking, dancing, running, cycling, swimming and so on. When this exercise is 'aerobic' it burns off calories, speeds up the body's metabolism, helps maintain a strong heart and may reduce the harmful type of cholesterol that can clog the arteries. It can also reduce fatigue. To be 'aerobic', it should leave the exerciser slightly breathless (*not* panting) and with an increased pulse (*not* a pounding heart). To be beneficial, it is thought to be important that the exercise is prolonged (20–30 minutes) and regular (at least three times a week). However, recent American studies indicate that a good result can also be obtained by splitting those 20 minutes into, say, five sessions of 4 minutes each. The GP should be consulted before embarking on a new exercise programme.

Forms of exercise popular with people with arthritis include the following:

■ **Walking** is a cheap, easy way to get fitter that can be readily incorporated into everyday life. Walking to the shops is much more relaxing than sitting in a traffic jam. People who use a walking stick can usually still benefit from walking unless they experience pain over very short distances.

■ **Dancing**, such as ballroom dancing or line dancing, is an excellent, enjoyable way to get exercise that improves mobility and balance.

■ **Swimming** is great all-round exercise, stretching and strengthening muscles as well as getting the heart going. The particular benefit of exercising in water is that it supports the body weight, enabling more exercise to be done. The Arthritis Research Campaign says that, for people with rheumatoid arthritis, learning to swim could be one of the best investments they make in their future.

■ **Hydrotherapy** is a common treatment for arthritis. The water is generally warmer than in the swimming pool, and exercise is under medical supervision. Ask the GP about local hydrotherapy facilities. Also look out for water-based exercise classes such as aquarobics – aerobics in the pool – or flotation aerobics. People with arthritis attending such classes should avoid straining to reach a position and must make sure that the teacher knows of their condition, as some movements may be inappropriate.

■ **Cycling** It's amazing how much modern cycles can be adapted to suit the individual's needs, while static exercise bikes are available for those who don't fancy the road. It is easy to prevent boredom while using an exercise bike by reading a book, listening to the radio or watching TV at the same time.

■ **Aerobics** There are specific classes aimed at people with disabilities and some have disabled aerobics instructors. High-impact classes where the feet hit the ground vigorously and often are not advised. People with arthritis will probably want to opt for low- or even no-impact exercise. Again, people with arthritis attending aerobics classes should avoid straining to reach a position and must make sure that the teacher knows of their condition, as some movements may be inappropriate.

■ **Sports** Golf, martial arts and t'ai chi, tennis and many other sports are enjoyed by people with arthritis. As always, consult your doctor before embarking on new activities.

Everyday activities, including vacuuming, dusting and cleaning the windows, also stretch the muscles, strengthen them and burn off calories. Approaching these activities with the same care and fore-thought as one would an exercise can help make them safer.

Exercise guidelines

■ Balance exercise with rest and relaxation.

■ Couple exercise with joint care. Avoid using heavy weights or staying in one position for too long. Kneeling and squatting, for example, should be avoided by anyone with knee problems.

■ Follow the two-hour rule – if more pain is felt two hours after exercising than before, less exercise should be done next time.

■ Little and often within a daily routine is best for ROM and for strengthening exercise.

■ It is best to exercise when pain and stiffness and tiredness are least and medication is having its maximum effect.

■ A warm bath or the application of heat (see pages 49–50 for some ideas) before more prolonged exercise may help relax the muscles.

Exercise has real benefits. It adds life to years and years to life.

It can be fun

Lucy

I call my favourite exercise "toelympics". Sit down, place a matchbox on the floor with the end up and try to pick it up with your bare toes. Not as easy as it sounds. As you become more proficient, try a mock game of noughts and crosses using alternate feet or even with an opponent!'

Especially with other disabled people

Catriona

'There was a real buzz in the room when we had a disabled aerobics instructor. I could see other people having problems keeping in time as well as me. We just smiled at one another and felt glad we weren't the only ones making a fool of ourselves. It didn't matter, though, because we were all having so much fun.'

And age is no barrier

Rita

'I'm in my 70s now but I am a new person, full of energy, free from any pain; and, to crown it all, my fourth hip operation became unnecessary. The muscles in my legs have become really strong and it seems that the hip joint has repaired itself. I can walk without pain – something that was denied me for 20 years. It is an understatement to say that exercise is good for you.'

For more *i*nformation

- *ⓘ* *Fit for Life: A Guide to Safe Exercises for People with Arthritis*, a free booklet from Arthritis Care (address on page 141).

- *ⓘ* *Alive and Kicking: The Carer's Guide to Exercises for Older People*, published by Age Concern Books (see page 155).

Diet

Diet is still probably the most controversial area in the treatment of arthritis. Some people make incredible claims about it; many doctors are still frankly sceptical. What is clear is that no diet will cure arthritis nor will one particular diet 'work' in all types of the disease.

This is not to say that the role of diet isn't important. If we are what we eat, then we might be able to alter what we are by altering what we eat. Any doctor will tell you that it is always a good idea to think about what you eat, and for people with arthritis it's worth thinking about a little more.

Joy

'I've discovered that citric acid [found in citrus fruit such as oranges and lemons, and artificially as flavouring E330] doesn't seem to agree with me so I try to keep that out of my diet. I don't know if it specifically affects my arthritis but I certainly feel better for avoiding it.'

From *Getting a Grip: Self-help for Arthritis and Rheumatism* by Jim Pollard (Headline 1996)

People with arthritis should certainly aim to eat a healthy diet:

- Eat a variety of food to get the full range of nutrients.
- Eat plenty of fruit and vegetables (ideally five portions a day).
- Eat plenty of foods rich in starch and fibre.
- Don't eat too much fat (especially saturated fats such as butter, meat fats).
- Don't eat sugary foods too often.
- Look after the vitamins and minerals when preparing your food.
- Drink plenty of fluids.
- Keep alcohol consumption within sensible levels.
- Aim to eat the right amount to be a healthy weight.

Eating a balanced diet should mean that mineral or vitamin supplements are unnecessary. However, for some people, including older people and those with disabilities, they may be appropriate. People with arthritis and osteoporosis should discuss their diet with their GP and ask if any supplements might be necessary.

What many people with arthritis want to know is whether there is anything beyond this that could help them. There are two areas worth considering: specialist dietary supplements and dietary manipulation. Neither has been researched in great depth

– certainly not to the satisfaction of most doctors – and most of the research that has been done has been on rheumatoid arthritis.

Common dietary supplements

Fish oils

The fatty acids in fish oil may produce less inflammatory chemicals than those from animal fats, suggesting that fish oil may ease joint pain and stiffness in inflammatory disease such as rheumatoid arthritis and lupus. According to the Arthritis Research Campaign, a recent study found that not only does cod liver oil reduce pain and inflammation in the joints of people with osteoarthritis but it also turns off the enzyme responsible for destroying cartilage. Fish oil is also good for your heart. However, fish oil takes three to six months to become effective and it needs to be taken long term despite the fact that long-term safety has yet to be investigated. Fish oils are not available on prescription but can be obtained from most pharmacist/chemist shops and health food shops.

Evening primrose oil

Evening primrose oil has effects similar to those of fish oils and takes as long to become effective. Fish oils and evening primrose oil can be taken together.

New Zealand green-lipped mussel

Extract of the New Zealand green-lipped mussel may have a mild anti-inflammatory effect, although evidence of its value in rheumatoid arthritis is limited.

Selenium

There is some evidence of a relationship between low levels of the trace element selenium and arthritis but it is not clear whether this can be remedied by a supplement. Selenium by mouth may be toxic in large quantities.

Iron

Anaemia in rheumatoid arthritis does not necessarily respond to iron supplements.

Garlic

Fresh garlic (rather than pearls) is good for the heart but its benefit in rheumatoid arthritis is not yet known.

There is no evidence that any of the supplements mentioned above is helpful in osteoarthritis, though this does not mean they are not in some cases. However, the most beneficial dietary treatment for osteoarthritis is to keep weight down (weight loss is discussed on page 48).

Glucosamine

This is a tablet sold as a health food, which means that it has not had the rigorous testing that would be needed to obtain a drug licence. It is a simple amino acid (a protein). There is a little medical research showing that it has a small effect of slowing the rate of deterioration of osteoarthritis. The recommended dose of 1500mg per day should be tried for at least three months. There is probably no additional benefit from chondroitin sulphate with which it is sometimes sold in combination.

Dietary manipulation

Dietary manipulation will work for only some people with rheumatoid arthritis – perhaps 40 per cent at most. It's a difficult process, which must be under a doctor's supervision to prevent the danger of malnutrition. It can also be disruptive to your life and needs a high level of commitment. If it doesn't work after six weeks, it is important to return to medical treatment to prevent joint damage. There are three stages:

■ **elimination** – removing pretty much all but a few simple foods from the diet;

- **reintroduction** – if symptoms disappear following elimination, foods are reintroduced one by one to see if they cause the symptoms to return; and
- **challenging** – removing and reintroducing what seem to be the problem foods to see if they really are the cause of the symptoms.

The challenging phase is particularly important because initial benefits may simply be the result of the natural ups and downs of rheumatoid arthritis or of the body responding to its starvation by producing more of its own corticosteroids or of a placebo response (discussed on page 56).

One form of arthritis in which changing the diet definitely does help is gout. Foods rich in purines (see the list on page 9) raise the level of uric acid in the blood and this is what causes gout. Fasting, however, can also bring on a gout attack.

Weight loss

Roughly four times our body weight goes through the joints in the lower limbs as we move around, so the less weight the less damage this can cause. An overweight person with osteoarthritis in the knees will benefit from losing weight. This may also be true for someone with osteoarthritis of the hips. Losing a few kilos can help reduce pain and disability.

Unfortunately, losing weight and maintaining the weight loss can be hard. Setting small but achievable monthly goals is often worth trying, perhaps enlisting the help of the GP or practice nurse, or joining a reputable slimming group. If necessary, get advice from the GP or a dietician about the foods to avoid and how to make sure that the overall diet is well balanced and nutritious.

For more *i*nformation

ⓘ *Food for Thought: A Guide to Diet and Arthritis*, a free booklet from Arthritis Care (address on page 141).

Pain control

The main symptom of arthritis is pain. Nearly everyone with arthritis experiences it frequently, while more than a third are in constant pain. This is unpleasant enough but pain can set up a vicious cycle of other problems: pain causes fatigue, which causes depression, which causes stress, which causes more pain. Reducing pain can break the cycle.

Pain control is a personal affair. We all need to mix and match to find what works for us, but it may help to talk to other people to find out how they manage their arthritis.

Rebecca

'I now have my own pain management programme. I take the painkillers I need, visit an osteopath and use heat and massage for pain relief. If walking hurts, I use my wheelchair and now I pay someone to do my housework instead of struggling on in pain. I keep my pain in place, and if something hurts I don't do it. There's nothing noble about suffering.'

From *Talk About Pain*, published by Arthritis Care

Scientists and pain control specialists have developed the idea of the 'pain gate'. This is located in the spinal cord, and closing it can prevent the nerve signals recognised as pain from ever reaching the brain. It can be closed both physically and mentally.

Three of the main ways of closing the pain gate are discussed elsewhere in this book (drugs – see pages 26–38; complementary therapies – see pages 55–66; and exercise – see pages 38–44) but there are others, discussed below.

Heat

Warmth messages can block pain messages by beating them to the pain gate. Applying heat also gets the blood flowing. That's why 'rubbing it better' – or a massage or a TNS machine (see below) – can really help. So can a hot bath, a hot towel, an electric blanket, nice thick sheets (eg flannel) or a hot water bottle (wrapped in a towel).

Heated pads may help. Some of these run off the mains, others use batteries or are heated in the microwave and some are operated with a special disc in the pad itself. Some have thermostats and a massage facility. They are available for various parts of the body but be careful: some are very expensive. Make sure that they are approved to BEAB (British) or CE (European) standards.

Cold

Applying cold numbs pain and, during a flare-up of symptoms, can reduce swelling and muscle spasms. Buy cold packs at the pharmacist/chemist shop or make them by wrapping a damp towel round a pack of frozen vegetables or a bag of crushed ice. Never apply ice direct to the skin. Stop when the affected area feels numb.

TNS (transcutaneous nerve stimulation)

Using a TNS machine involves small electrodes that are taped to the skin and gently vibrate. The minute electrical impulses help close the pain gate by providing an alternative stimulus. Make sure that they are approved to BEAB (British) or CE (European) standards. Some people love them; others find them useless. A lot depends on where the pain is.

Anyone with a pacemaker should *not* use TNS.

Joy

'I'm only on painkillers now because of the ulcer. I use a TNS machine which is extremely good but, because I have spinal arthritis, I can't bend my body enough to actually attach it to the affected parts – the daft thing is, of course, that it's particularly difficult on the days I really need it.'

From *Getting a Grip: Self-help for Arthritis and Rheumatism* by Jim Pollard (Headline 1996)

Occupying the mind

Keeping busy prevents the pain messages swarming around unhindered. This is why as full a life as possible really does help arthritis. But activity needs to be balanced with relaxation. To be most beneficial, relaxing should still occupy the mind. People can think about anything they like, provided they enjoy it. It could be what they will be doing in the future or something they did in the past. It may be family and friends or hobbies. Let the imagination roam free. Or they can try this simple relaxation technique:

■ Find a pleasant place where you won't be interrupted and there's nothing more than soft music in the background.
■ Sit comfortably, with head supported and eyes closed.
■ Breathe deeply, feeling your abdomen rise and fall.
■ Focus on your breathing.
■ Then think about a favourite place or journey – real or imaginary – or simply think calming words like love and peace.

For other, more focused, uses of the mind, explore meditation or hypnosis.

Sleep

A good night's sleep always helps but pain is usually at its worst from around 10pm, making it difficult to drop off. Altering sleep patterns and avoiding stimulants such as alcohol, cigarettes, tea or coffee in the couple of hours before going to bed might help. Or try a warm bath instead. Make sure that the bed is warm and comfortable (most people with arthritis prefer a firmer bed).

Nobody should feel guilty about taking themselves off to bed at times.

Trudi

'On bad days I indulge myself by watching morning TV in my dressing gown by the fire with a mug of tea. Or I might go to bed in the afternoon with a good book and a hot water bottle. This is part of the way I handle my pain.'

From *Talk About Pain*, published by Arthritis Care

Sex

Making love is one of the best ways of closing the pain gate and probably the most enjoyable one to try.

> ### Penny
>
> 'When it's shared with the one you love, sex is a great stress buster. Your awareness of pain may lessen because you are enjoying yourself. Enjoying making love with your partner will also boost self-esteem and help you stay in a positive frame of mind when tackling pain. It is very important to cherish and give attention to your body. Making love, gently and at a time appropriate to you, will have a healing effect. Choose positions that are comfortable. Be adventurous and experiment. Tell your partner what feels good. Sex is the best exercise you can get in a horizontal position, but never forget that cosy hugs and kisses are important too.'

Pain clinics

There are now pain clinics throughout the UK, many attached to hospitals. They were set up by anaesthetists and nurses and others to raise awareness of and meet the needs of people with pain. Some, but not all, are very good for people with arthritis.

For more *i*nformation

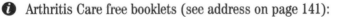

🛈 **NHS Direct** on 0845 46 47 can provide the address of the nearest pain clinic and is also a good first point of contact for finding out about NHS services.

🛈 Arthritis Care free booklets (see address on page 141):

Talk About Pain

Our Relationships, Our Sexuality.

Counselling

Counselling can certainly help in pain control. Unloading stress and negative emotions can break the pain cycle, which means that some people find that just talking about how they feel can take the pain away.

Seeking counselling is not a sign of not coping – either with arthritis or with the difficulties of caring or with life in general – rather the opposite. It is doing something about the things that are being troublesome.

Arthritis Care provides an excellent telephone helpline for people with arthritis and their carers. You can call on Freephone 0808 800 4050 or on 020 7380 6555. Counsellors may also be available through your GP, or they can be seen privately. Make sure they are registered with the British Association for Counselling and Psychotherapy (address on page 142). Fees are usually on a sliding scale depending on the person's resources. The advice on pages 57–59 on finding a complementary therapist you are comfortable with applies equally to counsellors.

Self-help groups

Talking with other people who have arthritis or with other carers can ease feelings of isolation, provide valuable information and support, and be a lot of fun. Arthritis Care has around 600 branches and local groups across the UK, aimed at people of all ages and from all sections of the community. Here are two happy Arthritis Care members.

Chris

'To be honest, I went along to be nosy and find out what they did. I found myself talking to everyone. It was very beneficial to be with other people in a similar position to myself, all having some form of arthritis. I felt comfortable with everyone. They were all so lovely and friendly that I assumed they'd all been meeting for years but, in fact, it was only the second get-together they'd ever had. The point is everyone understands the pain and frustrations I have felt. We have lots of laughs at these meetings, discussing our individual experiences of life.'

From *Talk About Pain*, published by Arthritis Care

Les

'It's not the individual activities that attract me to the group – the outings, the speakers and so on – although they are fun. It's the opportunity to talk to people who understand exactly what you're talking about without you having to explain the ins and outs of your problems. I find it supportive, informative and I get strength from it.'

There are also charities and support and self-help groups for people with specific types of arthritis. The more general ones are listed in the 'Useful addresses' section at the back of this book; for more specific groups, you can call the Arthritis Care helpline, see its magazine *Arthritis News* or ask in your local reference library for a directory of self-help groups.

Self-help groups also benefit carers.

Tom

'We've met a lot of interesting people and learned a lot from Arthritis Care. I met an occupational therapist at one meeting, who came round to assess the changes we needed to the house when my wife got arthritis. That sort of practical thing is happening all the time.'

For more *i*nformation

ⓘ **Arthritis Care** (address on page 141) produces useful booklets and provides information and support for people with arthritis and their carers.

ⓘ **Carers UK** has many local groups; contact the head office (address on page 143) for the one nearest you.

Complementary therapy

The term 'complementary therapy' covers a broad range of different treatments – from those generally accepted by the medical establishment, such as chiropractic and osteopathy, to those with no foundation in Western science at all. Some, like the two just mentioned, require the manipulation of the body. Others call for new skills to be learned, different lifestyles to be adopted or offer potions or pills. Some claim to work by faith alone. None will cure arthritis but they can help. Remember that no complementary treatment can undo joint damage that has already been done. People with arthritis will want to keep their doctors informed of any complementary therapies they are trying.

All the approaches have one thing in common: someone somewhere thinks they have helped them. There is probably one somewhere that can help most of us – including carers. The secret is to pick a way through the maze of complementary therapies to find the one(s) that suit the temperament and the bank balance as well as the medical condition.

Many of the complementary therapies listed in this chapter see the world and the human body within it in a different way from conventional medicine; their notions of research and evidence are not the same as those of Western scientists. Much evidence, for example, is anecdotal, based on people's reports of their own experience, rather than experimental. That does not, of itself, mean that these approaches do not work. Only that it is harder to prove. Sometimes the only way is a 'suck it and see' approach.

However, if a fair trial doesn't seem to have achieved anything, people should trust their judgement and move on.

Where pretty much all the complementary therapies differ from mainstream medicine is in what they aim to treat. Mainstream medicine treats the disease; complementary therapy treats the whole person, which immediately yields a benefit – the individual and their views are placed at the centre of the process. To someone with arthritis who is used to being treated like dozens of other similar patients with what can be considered a low-priority, long-term, unglamorous, marginalised condition, this will be enormously liberating.

In this person-centred or holistic approach the first session of most therapies is fairly long, perhaps an hour or even more, because the therapist will take a full personal and medical history. NHS doctors, even with the best will in the world, just do not have this sort of time.

Some doctors say that complementary therapy is just placebo – something that does nothing at all but helps a person who has faith in it. Placebos are used in trials to provide comparative data for the drug under scrutiny: half the people in the trial are given a placebo and the other half are given the new drug. Some of those who are given the placebo still get better. This is called the placebo effect, and some doctors dismiss complementary therapies as nothing more than this. Perhaps they are right. Who knows? But is that the most important issue? Most people are simply pleased that they have got better. Leave the scientists to worry about how. The placebo effect only serves to emphasise the power of the mind in health and healing.

The down-side of all this is obvious – anyone can claim anything will cure anything, and how are we to know whether they are telling the truth? There is only moderate regulation of the medical and health claims that people can make about themselves and their products. For example, some manufacturers blur the line between a food and a drug to maximise the health benefits they can claim for their products and minimise the regulations.

Some therapies have their own internal regulatory mechanisms and may have a list of registered practitioners who have reached certain standards or undergone certain periods of training. Some but not all. Choose a therapist carefully to minimise the chances of falling into the hands of an unscrupulous one.

The following sections mention some of the complementary therapies that are most popular with people with arthritis. Clearly, no one complementary therapy will work for everybody any more than any one medicine will, but, for people with arthritis, few are actually dangerous. Complementary therapies can help carers, too: you don't have to have a medical condition to benefit. Many of the therapies will simply make you feel good. Feelings of stress and difficulty relaxing or sleeping, for example, which are common in carers are also problems that complementary therapies are particularly good at helping you address.

Finding the right therapist

First, choose a therapy. Possible starters, to improve mobility in stiff (but not inflamed) joints, might be chiropractic, osteopathy or yoga. To reduce pain, consider acupuncture or reflexology. For a feel-good pick-me-up, try aromatherapy or massage.

Joy

'I also use aromatherapy. I read about it in a magazine and sent for the oils. My sister, who is a nurse, makes them up for me and other people with arthritis. I rub them into my skin two or three times a day. The effect doesn't last long but it's very soothing and smells lovely.'

From *Getting a Grip: Self-help for Arthritis and Rheumatism* by Jim Pollard (Headline 1996)

Second, approach the regulatory body for a list of local therapists (the Arthritis Care helpline or the local library can probably help here). Check just what inclusion on the list means. Does it signify certain qualifications or experience, or merely that a membership fee has been paid? For an unregulated therapy, try word of mouth. Begin with the most reliable sources, such as a GP or another health professional or therapist, before trying friends and relatives. Be very wary of the practitioner who approaches you direct, bearing a broad smile and a special introductory offer. A therapist's effectiveness is often in inverse proportion to the claims they make. Beware of somebody promising the Earth. The most likely result is that your therapy will end up costing it.

Third, ask questions. Before committing to anyone, however highly recommended, check them out.

■ What exactly do they do?
■ How long have they been doing it?
■ How did they start?
■ What training have they had? Where? For how long?
■ What professional bodies do they belong to?

A key question is whether they are insured. Few insurance companies will insure unqualified practitioners. Members of the Institute for Complementary Medicine should be insured through the Institute. No genuine therapist will mind questioning. After all, if theirs is a person-centred approach, it will be important to them that you feel comfortable.

Make sure you can talk to them. Do you understand what they are on about? Incomprehensible mystical mumbo-jumbo is of no use. Ask what their therapy will involve.

■ How long will each session take?
■ How long will the whole programme take?
■ What sort of benefits might you expect to see? When?

It is obviously important to ask how much it will all cost. Embarking on a programme that you cannot afford may create more problems than it solves. Explore these costs with your GP. The range of therapies to which a doctor can refer a patient is increasing all the time. Occasionally, a voluntary organisation may be able to help or perhaps there are sessions at a local authority leisure centre or other council facility.

Fourth, ensure that it is your choice. Don't be afraid to change your mind before starting or after a few sessions. Again, no genuine therapist will object. Don't be bullied into staying. If the therapist starts using language that suggests you are responsible for any failure or that makes you feel uncomfortable, head for the door. On the other hand, don't give up if results aren't immediate. Discuss your concerns with the therapist.

Fifth, get into it. Once in a consultation or session with a therapist, leave your scepticism behind. Go with what you have chosen to do and enjoy it. That way you maximise your chances of finding something that really helps.

Acupuncture

Acupuncture is recommended by its practitioners for pain relief, stress and sleep problems, and immune problems.

Basic principles Ancient Chinese. Acupuncture sees ill health as caused by imbalances in a body's energy (yin and yang). These can be corrected by stimulating the flow of healing chi energy at different acupoints on the body depending on the problem.

Methods of treatment Fine needles are inserted in the acupoints. Most people say it is not painful. As with most complementary therapies, the first session is usually a long one. The acupuncturist will be particularly interested in the client's reactions to the opposites of hot and cold, damp and dry, etc, asking what sort of food is preferred, what time of year and so on.

Length of treatment Three to six sessions are usually needed.

Attitudes of medical doctors Many doctors tend to accept that it can work for some people but suggest that, rather than chi energy, it is the body's natural painkilling endorphins that are stimulated by the needles. It may also increase the body's own release of corticosteroids.

Related therapies Acupressure and Shiatsu use a similar philosophical approach but with finger pressure instead of needles.

Regulatory body British Acupuncture Council (address on page 142).

Aromatherapy

Aromatherapy is recommended by its practitioners for respiratory problems, skin problems, chronic pain and anything in which stress is an element.

Basic principles Ancient Egyptian, Greek, Roman and Arab. Aromatherapy employs the healing properties of distilled oils from aromatic plants, called essential oils.

Methods of treatment It works primarily through the sense of smell but can often be combined with massage. The art, say practitioners, lies in choosing the right blend of oil for the right person at the right time. A good aromatherapy massage can be very relaxing indeed.

Length of treatment When required.

Attitudes of medical doctors Few would advise against it and most would acknowledge the benefits of massage and of stimulating the senses.

Regulatory body None. Look out for qualifications such as the Associate of Tisserand Aromatherapists (ATA) or membership of bodies such as the International Society of Practising Aromatherapists (ISPA) or the International Federation of Aromatherapists (IFA).

Chiropractic

Chiropractic is recommended by its practitioners for anything to do with the joints and muscles, including neck and back pain, headaches and tension.

Basic principles Developed by Canadian Daniel David Palmer in 1895, it focuses on the mechanical 'fixations' in the spine. Because this is the home of the central nervous system, these can cause problems throughout the body.

Methods of treatment 'Fixations' have many causes – injury, disease, allergy, stress or poor posture – and are treated by 'mobilisation' – moving the joint surfaces apart. This is done with the person lying on a couch, and most people say it is not painful.

Length of treatment Dealing with the initial problem may take only a handful of relatively short sessions but most chiropractors recommend regular visits.

Attitudes of medical doctors Generally positive, as the benefits of chiropractic can be demonstrated through research.

Regulatory body The British Chiropractic Association (address on page 142). The General Chiropractic Council (address on page 146) is a statutory body regulating chiropractic.

Western herbal medicine

Western herbal medicine – the forerunner of mainstream medicine – is recommended by its practitioners for most conditions, including arthritis, and particularly for stress, gastro-intestinal, menstrual and hormonal problems.

Basic principles The therapeutic use of herbs is as old as human beings. The Western tradition, which is based on Greek and Roman principles, sees the herbs as stimulating the body's healing process although many of their properties – anti-bacterial, anti-viral and so on – are much as mainstream synthetic drugs. Indeed, although herbal medicines are 'natural', they can be even more toxic than drugs so it is not a good idea to self-prescribe anything stronger than a herbal tea.

Methods of treatment Very full case histories are taken and often a physical examination is involved before a personalised herbal formula is prescribed.

Length of treatment One visit may be sufficient, although this is less likely with a complex condition such as arthritis.

Attitudes of medical doctors Not generally dismissive, as herbs are the basis of many modern drugs (eg aspirin contains a substance found in willow bark), but they tend to be concerned about the difficulties of getting a precise dose from a natural and therefore variable product. This is worth discussing with your herbalist.

Regulatory body The National Institute of Medical Herbalists (address on page 148). Look out for the initials MNIMH.

Chinese herbal medicine

Chinese herbal medicine is recommended by its practitioners for most conditions, including arthritis, for which, in China, it remains the most popular treatment even though Western medicine is now available there too.

Basic principles Chinese medicine, based on the principle of balance mentioned under acupuncture, is some 23 centuries old. It sees herbs – which are categorised according to their nature (eg hot or cold), taste and the particular organ they enter – as restoring the imbalances that cause disease.

Methods of treatment Pills or extracts are the most likely treatment for a chronic condition such as arthritis, and dietary suggestions may well be made. The approach is holistic, treating the whole person not just the problem presented.

Length of treatment More than one visit is likely to be needed, and, in general, treatments are slower acting than Western drugs.

Attitude of medical doctors Tend to be unenthusiastic despite the fact that some Chinese remedies have proved effective in trials. As with Western herbal medicine, there are concerns over getting a precise dose and occasional reports of serious ill-effects.

Regulatory body None, but many Chinese-trained practitioners are members of the Association of Traditional Chinese Medicine (address on page 142). Look out also for the Register of Chinese Herbal Medicine (RCHM).

Homeopathy

Homeopathy is recommended by its practitioners for most conditions, although homeopaths would suggest an osteopath or chiropractor for structural problems.

Basic principles Founded by the German doctor Samuel Hahnemann in the eighteenth century, it is based on the principle that like cures like. An immeasurably small amount of the substance that causes the problem is used to stimulate the body's own healing mechanisms.

Methods of treatment A detailed personal history will be taken. Medicines – usually a single remedy – are generally given in small sugary tablets.

Length of treatment Sessions may be long, especially the first one. With a chronic condition such as arthritis, several sessions over some time may be required.

Attitudes of medical doctors Homeopathy is available on the NHS, and there is research to suggest that it does work in some cases. However, nobody can explain satisfactorily why it works, given that the dilutions in the dose are so great that, according to the laws of physics, the original is no longer measurably present.

Regulatory body There are two, the Society of Homeopaths and the British Homeopathic Association (addresses on page 149 and page 142). Members of the latter organisation are also trained doctors.

Massage

Massage is recommended by its practitioners for anybody at all, and specifically for aches and pains related to stress and muscle tension.

Basic principles We all know the benefit of touch. That's why we rub the spot when we hurt ourselves. Massage helps eliminate toxins, stimulate the flow of blood and lymph, and soothe the nerves. There are two types: remedial and relaxation.

Methods of treatment The client will be asked what sort of massage is required – vigorous and stimulating or gentle and relaxing – and if any parts of the body are to be avoided (eg an inflamed joint). Clothes are removed and towels used to cover the body. These are removed and replaced as each part of the body is worked on – the masseur rubbing, kneading and stimulating the body as required. Massage is often combined with aromatherapy, and all masseurs will use oils or talcum powder. A massage must be stopped if it is painful.

Length of treatment As required; massage is a feel-good treatment rather than a remedy.

Attitudes of medical doctors Positive, so long as it's done carefully. Some hospitals now make massage available to patients.

Regulatory body None, although lists of qualified masseurs and aromatherapy masseurs are available from the Institute for Complementary Medicine (address on page 146).

Osteopathy

Osteopathy is recommended by its practitioners for anything structural, including arthritis.

Basic principles Founded in 1874 by American doctor Andrew Taylor Still, a Christian who believed that if we are created in God's image then all faults in our functioning must arise from the way we use our bodies. Osteopaths attempt to right these misalignments to allow the bodily fluids and nerves to work correctly.

Methods of treatment The person lies on a couch while the osteopath makes 'adjustments' and relaxes the soft tissues to allow the body to heal itself. Most people find it relaxing and not painful.

Length of treatment This will depend on the problem. With arthritis, regular visits may be suggested. The osteopath will usually say how many treatments will be needed to achieve a result.

Attitudes of medical doctors Generally positive, as they are for chiropractic.

Regulatory body The General Osteopathic Council (address on page 146).

Reflexology

Reflexology is recommended by its practitioners for anybody, but particularly for aches and pains, immune system problems, stress and lack of energy.

Basic principles There are indications that there was something like reflexology in ancient Eastern cultures but its modern father is American ear, nose and throat specialist William H Fitzgerald. He discovered that pressure applied to one part of the body could relieve pain in another. Using this principle, a reflexologist accesses the whole body – which is divided into zones – from the foot. Massage here can unblock energy flows between zones and promote healing.

Methods of treatment Pressure with the practitioner's thumb to the person's foot and sometimes hand. It's too firm to tickle but may be slightly painful as 'blockages' are released. Most people feel good after a treatment.

Length of treatment Perhaps once every six weeks or so.

Attitudes of medical doctors Most acknowledge the benefit of a foot massage although few accept reflexology's full analysis. Physiotherapists and occupational therapists are usually more enthusiastic.

Regulatory body None, but the largest independent organisation is the Association of Reflexologists (address on page 142). The initials MAR indicate that the therapist has a qualification in reflexology.

Yoga

Yoga is recommended by its practitioners for anybody to improve posture, muscle tone and flexibility and to help relaxation.

Basic principles Ancient Eastern, particularly Indian. The various positions (or asanas) adopted in yoga have evolved over thousands of years. By moving the body in different ways and directions they stimulate muscles and joints and help the circulation and the flow of bodily fluids.

Methods of treatment Yoga is not strictly a therapy, because nobody practices on anyone. Many books are available, but the best way to learn the asanas and the breathing and meditation techniques that can accompany them is from a teacher. Classes are run at most adult education and leisure centres. People with arthritis should avoid straining to reach a position and must make sure that the teacher knows of their condition, as some positions may be inappropriate. A therapeutic yoga teacher may be able to provide a customised programme.

Attitudes of medical doctors Be careful with your joints.

Regulatory body There are many types of yoga and no single regulatory body.

Other therapies

Where no governing body is listed, or for information on other therapies, contact the Institute for Complementary Medicine (address on page 146).

For more *i*nformation

ⓘ The Arthritis Care booklet *The Balanced Approach: A Guide to Medicines and Complementary Therapies* looks at the most popular complementary therapies for people with arthritis (address on page 141).

ⓘ *Know Your Complementary Therapies*, published by Age Concern Books (see page 155).

3 What should you do?

This chapter discusses frankly the challenges that caring brings, and aims to help you decide what best to do. It looks at what it is like to be cared for, whether you should consider becoming a carer and what rights you will have if you do.

Sheena

'Last year we were given a shop for the day for Carers UK at our local shopping mall. We made lots of posters – all by hand – and put them in the shop. We went there first thing in the morning, started putting balloons up and getting ready, and when we looked there was a queue right the way down the shopping mall of people waiting to come in.

'They couldn't wait for us to open, to ask all these questions. It was incredible. You can't believe the people who are out there. It was carers listening to other carers. Some carers are frightened to go and talk to anybody official. They feel that they might lose their pensions or their little bit of money, or the help that they've got. But they were only too happy to come in and discuss it with us. Because really – let's face it – we, other carers, are the true professionals.'

Are you a carer already? Carers UK uses the following simple definition:

'Carers look after family, partners or friends in need of help because they are ill, frail or have a disability. The care they provide is unpaid.'

It's easy to slide along the scale – a few hours become a few more hours become a few days. This may well be the right way for you to go but it is important to do it with your eyes open. When you are considering what you should do for your relative or friend or partner with arthritis, the first thing to think about is: what is it like to be cared for?

What is it like to be cared for?

There is no doubt that being a carer can be hard work. But being cared for also has its problems and frustrations.

Maria

'It's not easy being "cared for". It's not just the messy bits. It's no longer being able to nick a chocolate biscuit out of the fridge, or experiment with make-up, or grab just the right scarf to set off your jumper as you rush out the door. Always, always, you have to ask.

'These things may seem insignificant nit-pickings compared with the more obviously dramatic changes wrought by disability, but taken together they are momentous. As they are given up, a little bit of what outwardly makes you an individual is eroded.

'No one would deny that looking after another person can be tough. It is also often a job reluctantly undertaken. Knowing all this, reading all the accounts of ruined lives, it can be just as tough finding yourself in the position of having to receive all this "care" – your self-esteem can easily be drowned out by guilt and gratefulness. If carers are way down the ladder then those they care for are at the bottom, popularly seen as tyrants, as indifferent to their helper's feelings as pampered pet poodles.'

What is caring?

'Caring' is a nice word – we all like to think we care – but it's tough work emotionally, physically and financially. Just what are you taking on if you become someone's carer?

It is important to distinguish between caring *about* and caring *for*. Caring about each other has got to be a good thing – the world needs more of it. Caring for someone is more complicated. It's what we do for those who can't do it for themselves. To be cared for is something that all adults need and enjoy from time to time but few would want *all* of the time. And most people with arthritis probably don't. So you need to bear this fact in mind: if you choose to become another adult's carer you are becoming something they would rather not have. For this reason it should be a fall-back position – a plan B (or even plan C, D or E) – rather than a first choice. If you care about someone (in the first sense of the word), you'll want to give them what we all want: as much independence as possible for as long as possible.

Be clear what being a carer involves. Many carers provide personal help with toileting and bathing, for example, and with physically demanding tasks such as lifting and washing. In the case of arthritis, there can also be a lot of small but frequent tasks such as opening bottle tops or turning taps on or off. The 2001 Census indicates that 1.25 million carers care for more than 50 hours a week. Figures quoted by Crossroads show that as many as two-thirds of carers say that their own health has suffered as a result of their caring responsibilities.

It is estimated that carers save the State around £57 billion a year. However, it is work that is seldom recognised by the rest of us and certainly not adequately by the State. Listen to Hilary, who cares for a friend with fibrositis.

Hilary

'I would like to see carers who are looking after a relative or friend accorded the same financial and professional treatment as the social services provide care assistants. If you're a carer on Income Support or Pension Credit you may get a premium but it's just £25 a week compared to £5 an hour for a care assistant. Getting grants is harder, too. Some applications need a social worker's recommendation but if you're a private carer you might not have a social worker. This is my second time as a carer and it's harder the second time around because you know more about what you may have to do and you know how little help you're going to get to do it. If official bodies know what a carer is, you're lucky – although this is improving now.'

The concern with money isn't penny-pinching. It's reality for many carers. Fifty per cent of carers give up work to provide care, according to Carers UK. And it can be a full-time job.

Hilary again

'It's not easy to switch off. You don't have your own life unless the person you're caring for is out of the house or with someone you trust. Otherwise, every second, you're aware of what they're doing. If the person you care for can't go out much, neither can you.

'I'm fortunate to be on the Internet so I can 'go out' from inside my own home. I monitor a carers' newsgroup but I also use it to talk about other things. It stops me feeling alienated from the world. I think it's that alienation that non-carers find hard to understand. The thing is that, when you love the person you're caring for, you can't just walk away. How do you turn round and say "I'm sorry, I can't cope with you"?'

In short, caring involves giving a lot. Some people are better suited temperamentally to this than others; some are even attracted to it, and the system certainly relies on this. However, if you give up your own life for another, you are not necessarily doing them a favour. If your own health breaks down, you will no longer be able to provide them with the same service while at the same time their guilt and resentment will grow – guilt over what you're doing for them and the damage it is doing to you and resentment over the degree of control you have over their lives. You may feel guilt and resentment too – guilt over what you are not doing for them and resentment over what you do.

If you doubt that this will happen to you, think seriously about why you are considering becoming a carer. Is it because you feel sorry for the other person? Is it a sense of duty? Is it out of love? All three probably, if you're honest with yourself. Duty and sympathy, even if tempered with the strongest of love, can conjure up guilt and resentment sooner or later. You should not feel bad about the negative feelings you will at times have towards the person for whom you care. Sometimes they'll be very strong. And don't kid yourself that you won't have them, because you will not find a carer who hasn't had them at some point. Better to have thought about it and, ideally, have talked about it in advance. Better still to have explored options for independence and professional caring first.

Control is a key issue. Caring should be a supportive role, not a decision-making one. For this reason, many disabled people prefer the term 'personal assistant' to 'carer', because this term makes it far clearer where the decisions are made. You are there to help the person you are caring for to live the life they want to, not to decide what sort of life that should be. This can be very difficult because they will, at some point, make a decision that you don't like or agree with. That much is guaranteed.

If you do become a carer, it is important that you have an outlet for the negative feelings you will experience. You don't want to take them out on the person you are caring for but you must not bottle them up.

Caroline

'I was caring for my husband, Jeff (who had arthritis), working full-time as a teacher and bringing up a son. I had no relatives and felt it was all on my shoulders. I felt very responsible. The inevitable happened. My job became so stressful that I took early retirement, my asthma was terrible and I was diagnosed with depression. I saw a counsellor and it was she who pointed out just what I was taking on. The thing is I was feeling guilty about my negative feelings, which was no good. You have to let them out or you'll get depressed. You're not a horrible person for having horrible feelings. If you feel angry, it's because you've got a lot to be angry about. Look after yourself.

'Before Jeff died, I apologised for all the harsh things I'd said to him and he said he understood. As a carer, you don't just need information, you need support – from other carers and, I think, from a professional counsellor – a safe confidential place where you can say all those things you're ashamed about feeling.'

So, before getting into the ins and outs of everyday caring, it's important to have a clear idea of your role as a carer. The needs of the person you are caring for must be your focus. That means the needs they express, not the needs you believe they have. Of course, if the person's health prevents them from expressing their needs then that is a different situation but this is not the case with a physical disability such as arthritis.

This means that your relationship with the person should be such that they feel comfortable about expressing their true feelings with you, and you with them. Few relationships enjoy that degree of frankness – we often, for the best of motives, protect the ones we love from our real feelings. It's far easier to be blunt with a professional carer. A relationship will change when one party begins to care for (rather than care about) the other. It has to. It will challenge even the most loving relationship.

Jenny

'I was still at school when Mum first got bad, and the role reversal was very stressful. It affected my exams. Helping with personal tasks is tough for us both. I feel that her loss of dignity is in some ways worse for her because I'm her daughter.

'My advice is to get help as soon as possible. Mum has an occupational therapist now who helps a lot with equipment and a home help three times a week, but she's really had to fight for everything.'

If you become a carer, it must be your choice. There are alternatives, as this book will show. 'I *had* to' is not a good enough reason – you owe it to yourself and the person you are caring for to have thought about it more thoroughly than that.

My mum says that my grandfather used to say to her 'You only have children so they can look after you in your old age', and he was only partly joking. It was clear what he expected and, in due course, she did look after him. She has made it equally clear that she doesn't expect the same from me or my brother – not least because of the difficulties it caused her. So ideas of family obligation vary with our own upbringing and attitude – they are not fixed. You do *not* have to do it.

Think creatively. Maximise the options that maintain the other person's independence, rather than helping them too much. In truth, the best carer may not be someone with the traditional caring skills but someone who is assertive and knows their rights and those of the person they are caring for. The health service and local and central government do have caring roles and responsibilities – the best service you can give may be to ensure that these roles and responsibilities are taken.

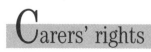

Carers' rights

However clearly you see your role as a carer (and it is important that you *do* see it clearly), your role in the eyes of the state and society in general will probably be unclear. Some people still see caring as the natural extension of a family relationship, and for a long time governments have thought the same.

When he was piloting through Parliament the Private Member's Bill that became the *Carers (Recognition and Services) Act 1995*, Malcolm Wicks was blunt about how carers are seen by themselves and others. He said that carers are:

'taken for granted by the welfare state, taken for granted by social workers and doctors, and not given the support that they need. Often the GP or the social worker visiting is almost literally patting the person on the back, saying: "You're doing a great job, keep going". Instead of saying: "Hang on a minute, how are you? When did you last have a good night's sleep? When did you have a break? Is there anything we can do for you?" And that's the mentality that we've got to change round.'

Section 8 of the *Disabled Persons Act 1986* says that when assessing disabled people for services under Section 2 of the *Chronically Sick and Disabled Persons Act 1970*, local authorities *must* take account of the carer's ability to provide care on a regular basis.

You can ask for your own care needs to be assessed when the person you care for is being assessed or reassessed. (Assessments are covered in detail on pages 86–90.) This right is set out in *The Carers (Recognition and Services) Act 1995* and applies to anyone who provides, or intends to provide, a substantial amount of care on a regular basis. The *Carers and Disabled Children Act 2000* extends this right, giving carers the right to have their needs assessed even if the cared-for person does not want an assessment.

A carer may themselves be found to have community care needs and to be entitled to community care services in their own right, but the type of help that can be given is not limited to community care services. For example, if the person who is being cared for refuses to accept help from anyone but a relative, the local authority might provide the relative with help with housework so that they had free time to help their relative. However, these services cannot include services providing personal or intimate care. If the carer and the cared-for person both agree, the local authority can also provide services to the carer instead of providing community care services for the cared-for person but, again, these cannot include intimate care services. In England and Wales carers can now also receive direct payments to enable them to purchase care themselves (see pages 90–91). These are available as an alternative to both community care services and to non-community care services provided under the *Carers and Disabled Children Act 2000*.

In Scotland a carer is entitled to an assessment of their needs which will be taken into account in deciding the services the person being cared for is offered.

For further *i*nformation

i Perhaps the best source of further information on this is other carers, particularly those among your friends and family whom you can talk to honestly about your concerns and those in your area who can advise you of what is available locally. Contact **Carers UK** (address on page 143).

i Age Concern Factsheets (see page 157 for details of how to obtain factsheets):

6 *Finding Help at Home*

24 *Direct Payments from Social Services*

41 *Local Authority Assessment for Community Care Services.*

4 Who can help?

The most important person in the management of arthritis is the person who has it. Nevertheless, there are a whole range of other people it is sensible to involve, the most obvious being the health professionals.

This chapter outlines where you can go for help – health and social services professionals, voluntary organisations and the family. Also discussed are suggestions for getting the best out of them. Making sure that service providers are aware of your needs and those of the person you are caring for is a key part of the challenge.

Caroline

'The GP is your gateway to local authority and other support. Try to find a GP who understands your role. Be honest with your GP. State what you need, don't wait for it to be offered, and keep asking.'

General practitioner (GP)

Everybody has the right to be registered with a GP – the first port of call for any illness, including a carer's.

Finding a GP

It has been estimated by Arthritis Care and the Arthritis Research Campaign that at least one in five GP appointments concerns arthritis, so a good relationship between a person with arthritis and their GP is very important. Similarly, make sure your own GP knows all about your caring responsibilities, so it will be easier for them to notice if these affect your health. It is possible that you too have some arthritis yourself, so take this opportunity to learn about managing it effectively. Don't wait until the condition becomes a serious problem.

When you register with a new GP, you should be offered an introductory health check. This should be repeated annually for patients who are 75 or over. If it is not offered, ask. Also ask for information about the services the practice offers and for a copy of the practice leaflet. This should outline what you can expect from the practice: opening times, facilities for disabled people and children, arrangements for tests and repeat prescriptions, and so on.

People with arthritis tend to need the assistance of a broad range of health professionals, so the more services a GP practice can provide – physiotherapy, counselling, practice nurse and so on – the better. A 'one-stop shop' makes referral easier and reduces travelling. Familiarity enables better relationships to be built. For this reason a larger multi-doctor practice or health centre is probably your best bet.

Everyone living in the UK has a right to register with a GP. You can choose your doctor, providing that they agree to accept you – you may be unable to register with the local GP of your choice if they may already have too many patients, for example. If you want to change your GP, go to the practice of your choice and ask to be registered, taking your medical card with you if possible. Lists of GPs are available from your local Primary Care Trust (the address will be in the telephone directory or available from the local library) or from NHS Direct on 0845 46 47. Details are also available on the NHS website www.nhs.uk by entering your town or postcode.

It could be worth trying to find a GP who is a member of the Primary Care Rheumatology Society, an organisation for family doctors with a special interest in arthritis. Ask your GP whether they are a member. If they are not, encourage them to join.

Remember that most carers have, or develop, their own health problems. Don't ignore them. You need to take care of yourself if you are to take care of someone else. See your own GP sooner rather than later if you have any problems.

What can the GP offer?

Many people with arthritis feel that there is little that a GP can do for them. This is not so. GPs monitor drugs, suggest other forms of treatment and advise on exercise, diet and anything else the patient might like to try.

In most cases of arthritis, the GP will be up against a disease that is difficult to diagnose, affects different people in different ways and for which there are treatments but no cures. A tough challenge. Time is an important factor in the diagnosis of arthritis but the symptoms such as pain, swelling and fatigue need immediate treatment. So, a prescription without a full explanation may well be the initial response. That's all right at first but don't put up with it for too long.

Referral

A very important thing that a GP can do is provide a referral to specialists. Joint pain is the biggest single reason for referral to hospital, so a request should not be refused. In 2004 the waiting time is set to be under 13 weeks. By 2005 GPs will be able to book appointments online. They will also be able to offer patients more choice of where they are referred – more hospitals, including private and continental hospitals.

Nobody is obliged to see a consultant – many people with arthritis manage their disease with their GP alone – but it makes sense to take advantage of a specialist's greater knowledge and hospital facilities. Anybody whose arthritis is sufficiently severe that they have care needs that can only be met by someone else should see a consultant. Everyone with suspected rheumatoid arthritis, ankylosing spondylitis or vasculitis (inflamed blood vessels) should press to see a consultant, even if this means travelling some distance.

Hospital consultant

Hospital consultants who specialise in arthritis and rheumatic diseases are called rheumatologists. Although they will use many of the diagnostic techniques discussed in Chapter 2, they will know more about the disease than a GP and be more familiar with its many variations. The consultant rheumatologist is usually the leader of a team that will take overall responsibility for treatment. They may also refer on to another health or community professional or, in some cases, to an orthopaedic surgeon who specialises in joint replacement and other surgery.

The Royal College of Physicians estimates that there should be one rheumatologist for every 85,000 people. The NHS falls some way short of this. For this reason it can take a long wait and possibly a long journey to see a rheumatologist. Nurses are taking on more and more work from doctors, however, and there are many nurse specialists/practitioners now employed by rheumatology departments.

Surgery

Operations for arthritis include joint replacement, joint fusion, removal of inflamed tissue, removal of some bone to ease pain, repair of damage to tendons, and release of a trapped nerve.

Replacements are usually offered if the joint has become very badly damaged and is not responding to other treatment. The most common is a hip replacement, although knees, ankles, shoulders, elbows and joints in the wrists and fingers can also be replaced. The joint is removed under anaesthetic and replaced with an artificial one, called a prosthesis, made from plastic and metal. All prostheses have to meet a European standard, although testing is still not as rigorous as for a new drug.

Over 50,000 hips are replaced every year in the UK. The vast majority of hip replacements leave the patient without pain and with three-quarters of 'normal' mobility in the joint. A modern prosthesis can last 15 years or more but should be checked regularly using X-ray and physical examination. Some 10–20 per cent of hip replacements are 'revisions' (ie repeat operations). Knees are the second most commonly replaced joint.

Replacements used to be 'saved' for patients over 60 but now younger people are also likely to be offered one. Surgery is not inevitable in arthritis but it can revolutionise a person's quality of life. Someone whose arthritis is sufficiently severe that they have care needs that can only be met by somebody else is the sort of patient who is more likely to be offered surgery or, indeed, to ask for it. It's always the patient's choice to proceed.

The key questions when considering surgery are:

- What exactly is being offered?
- What are the benefits?
- What should be possible afterwards that is not possible now?
- What will not be possible?
- What are the risks? (These are small but include infection, thrombosis, dislocation of the joint and, in a very tiny number of cases, death.)
- Who will do the surgery and what experience do they have?
- What prosthesis will be used and what is its track record like?

Surgeons are not robots. Some are better than others. A surgeon who performs a specific operation once or twice a year is unlikely to be as experienced, and therefore as competent, as a surgeon who performs the same procedure 30 times. Common sense suggests that the more common a type of surgery, the greater the likelihood that the surgeon performing it is experienced, but it makes sense to talk to your surgeon about their record and expertise as well as with other patients, friendly doctors, the theatre sister or the relevant business manager in the hospital.

It is extremely valuable to talk to someone else who has had the operation. Such people may be found through the hospital but the best bet is probably a local group of Arthritis Care or a local disability organisation. Arthritis Care produces a booklet about how best to prepare for and recover from the operation. Called *Surgery: A Guide for People with Arthritis*, the booklet details the most commonly performed operations and gives useful information. Hospitals often provide this too, but the standard of their written information sometimes falls far below that recommended by the Arthritis and Musculoskeletal Alliance (ARMA).

Kate Llewelyn was 25 when she had her knee replaced. She told *Arthritis News:*

Kate

'It has been ten months since my operation and I can't stop raving about my knee. It is amazing – free of pain and it bends to over 95 degrees.'

But it's not plain sailing.

Kate again

'The first week post-op was not pleasant. The painkilling regimen made me very ill and didn't work. My saviours were the physiotherapists, despite the weeks of pain they put me through. It was they who made my new knee work.'

Author Leslie Thomas has had both hips replaced. He says quite simply that they've changed his life.

Leslie

'It knocked the stuffing out of me for six months but it was the best thing I've ever done and I'd have no hesitation about doing it again. The only thing is, I still can't get out of the bath. I play cricket again now, a couple of sets of tennis, although I can't walk far enough to play golf.'

81

Hip replacement and other surgical waiting times are supposed to be under 12 months. Patients Choice runs the National Waiting List Helpline (Freephone 0800 032 9191) which can sometimes help patients find a shorter waiting list than the one they have been referred to.

Hip replacements can be carried out privately. If you are tempted by this option, don't be swayed by niceties such as a private room or an exotic menu; check out the things that really matter. Ask about the experience and expertise of the surgeon very carefully. If you will be in a private hospital, ask about the quality and amount of nursing care, and what will happen if anything goes wrong. Don't assume that private health care will get you better treatment than on the NHS.

For more *i*nformation

ⓘ Arthritis Care booklet *Surgery: A Guide for People with Arthritis* (address on page 141).

Physiotherapist (physio)

A patient can be referred for physiotherapy by their GP or consultant, or can pay for it privately. Some larger GP practices may have a visiting physiotherapist. Otherwise, it may be necessary to attend the hospital physiotherapy department. For physiotherapy, it is unlikely that referral will be to any hospital other than the local one but it doesn't hurt to ask.

Hospital physiotherapists are usually generalists rather than specialists. For the more common forms of arthritis with 'typical' mobility problems they should be fine. Otherwise, it can sometimes be a bit of a lottery. Quality and expertise vary within departments, so it can be worth asking to see someone with experience of the specific type of arthritis.

Having the 'right' physiotherapist is important because their work is often crucial in the treatment of arthritis. They concentrate on relieving pain and improving mobility of the joints using manipulation and treatments such as ultrasound (which stimulates the body tissue using inaudible, high-frequency sound waves), ice-packs and heat. They will probably suggest exercises to be done at home, most of which might seem so simple that it can be difficult to believe that they will work. In fact, they are highly effective and well worth the effort.

A typical course of treatment will last about ten sessions. Most hospitals are reluctant to offer longer term care because of the cost. For a long-term condition such as arthritis, this is not helpful.

Private physiotherapy is worth considering for more specialised or intensive help. For names of local private physiotherapists, contact the Chartered Society of Physiotherapy (see address on page 143). See only a physiotherapist who is a member of the Society and who understands both arthritis in general and the needs of the person you are caring for in particular.

In some areas, hydrotherapy may be available. This is physiotherapy in the water, done under the supervision of physiotherapists. Most people find that it helps their arthritis and virtually everyone enjoys it. The hydrotherapy pool is lovely and warm, and special equipment (such as lifting devices) is available so that even the most severely disabled people can benefit.

Joy

'I used to do hydrotherapy every week for about 20 minutes. A senior physiotherapist helped with the exercises. It's amazing how much exercise you can do in the lovely warm water that you can't do on land. The problem is that it's not available everywhere on the NHS; even where it is, it's usually only for a short time. Our Arthritis Care group hired the hydro pool so we could all go regularly – we took 30 to 40 people.'

From *Getting a Grip: Self-help for Arthritis and Rheumatism* by Jim Pollard (Headline 1996)

Occupational therapist (OT)

The occupational therapist is a health professional a carer really needs to know about, because they can make a real difference and may become a long-term ally for you and the person you are caring for. An occupational therapist will discuss with the person with arthritis their day-to-day activities, and can then advise about any aids or gadgets that might be helpful or even suggest structural alterations to the home. It is very important to tell the occupational therapist about what cannot be done – it is surprising how many difficulties can be overcome with a little imagination. Sometimes the occupational therapist may be limited to merely making recommendations, so you may have to do some lobbying as well to get them implemented.

The objective is to enable the person with arthritis to do as many everyday tasks as possible, as easily as possible while protecting their joints as much as possible. Simply rearranging the home or adjusting the way something is gripped or lifted may make a significant difference – and at no cost.

Occupational therapists work either as part of the hospital rheumatology team or for the social services. Those based in the hospital usually do splinting and arrange for the loan of equipment to be used at home; those from social services are generally concerned with a person's coping abilities and can recommend household equipment such as rising chairs, ramps and stairlifts. Social services occupational therapists are usually contacted by referral from the doctor; sometimes, though, from reluctance, ignorance or absent-mindedness, doctors may not refer as often as they could. Insist. Alternatively, contact one through your social services department. (There is more about social services on page 86.)

For more *i*nformation

ⓘ Arthritis Care booklet *Reaching Independence: A Guide to Living at Home for People with Arthritis* gives more information about OTs (address on page 141).

Pharmacist

Pharmacists can give advice about the medicines that the person you care for needs, whether they are on prescription or bought over the counter. Although you can use any pharmacy you wish, it may be helpful to use one regularly and to get to know the pharmacist. Some pharmacist/chemist shops have a prescription collection and delivery service or they may make home visits. Many have a computer database that can print out information about any specific drug or maintain computerised patient medication records, which detail the medicines dispensed for individual patients.

Helping someone get the best out of a health professional

■ Ask the person you are caring for if they would like you to accompany them to an appointment, and respect their right to say 'no'.

■ If you do go together, offer practical support such as taking notes or running a cassette recorder.

■ Discuss beforehand what they hope to get out of the appointment and what specific questions they want answered. Gently remind them of these during the consultation if necessary.

■ Discuss with them how they will answer the more obvious questions but do not, during the consultation, answer for them. Resist any attempts the professional might make to talk to you rather than the patient.

■ Try to encourage the person you are caring for to say more if you feel they are trivialising their arthritis or worrying about wasting the professional's time. Encourage the professional to say more if they are not speaking plainly.

■ Talk to health professionals as you would a genuine friend, even if they don't feel like one.

■ Arthritis Care produces good practice guidelines for primary health care (GPs, etc) and secondary health care (hospitals). Make sure the health professionals you deal with have copies.

Kate Lorig, Director of Patient Education Research at Stanford Arthritis Center in the USA, believes that the good patient should be a CAD: 'Come prepared. Ask questions. Discuss problems.' This technique can be applied equally well to your appointments with all health professionals or complementary therapists.

For more *i*nformation

ⓘ Age Concern Factsheet 44 *NHS Services and Older People* (see page 157 for details of how to obtain factsheets).

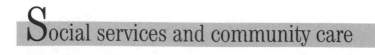

Social services and community care

There are various Acts of Parliament under which local authorities can provide or arrange community care services, notably the *NHS and Community Care Act 1990*. Two Acts specifically give people who are disabled the right to social services – the *Chronically Sick and Disabled Persons Act 1970* (CSDP Act) and the *Disabled Persons (Services, Consultation and Representation) Act 1986*.

The CSDP Act requires councils to make arrangements for the provision of certain services to individual chronically sick and disabled people in their area if they are necessary to meet the needs of the person. The services are:

■ practical assistance within the home;
■ disability aids and equipment;
■ assistance with adaptations to the home;
■ provision of meals at home or elsewhere;
■ help with installing or adapting a telephone;
■ help with taking advantage of educational or recreational facilities, including help with transport; and
■ provision of holidays.

A disabled person can ask for their needs to be assessed under the *Disabled Persons Act 1986* and must be provided with services under the CSDP Act if they are needed. In addition, the *Community Care (Direct Payments) Act 1996* gives local authorities the power to give disabled people direct payments so that they can buy their own care (see below).

Your relative does not need to be registered as disabled to receive services under these Acts but they have to fit the definition of 'substantially and permanently handicapped'. Anybody whose arthritis is so severe that they have care needs should be covered by this definition.

In practice, the degree of help given is limited by the resources available. However, the statutory obligation remains, creating what can be a complex legal situation. If you feel harshly or unfairly treated, don't give up. Read this section carefully and then reapply, appeal or take further advice.

Community care is co-ordinated through the local authority's social services department. In most parts of England and Wales, social services comes under the county council or unitary authority; in London it is the metropolitan or borough council. In Scotland the social work department is under the regional council, and in Northern Ireland social services comes under the local health and social services board or trust. Under the new Single Assessment Process for Older People (SAP) an assessment for social services is combined with health needs.

Getting the best out of a community care assessment

The first step is to make an appointment with the social services department for an assessment to determine 'needs'. They have an obligation to assess:

- anyone who is disabled;
- anyone who helps to look after someone else – in which case both people's needs should be assessed; and
- anyone else who 'appears to need' services.

The local authority must assess anyone with any need for a service which it has the power to provide (ie those listed on page 86), even if it does not provide that service at the time. A reassessment should be requested whenever a person's needs change.

Each local authority has its own assessment procedure. Ask to see its long-term care charter called *Better Care, Higher Standards* which explains its procedures, including such information as how long one should have to wait for an assessment. The assessment – which is free – should be carried out by a social worker, occupational therapist, social services care manager, community nurse or other professional but there is no national standard. The assessment interview can take place in the person's home, in hospital or in a council office. The person being assessed can have a friend or relative with them; this is a good idea for moral support and to act as an aide memoire.

Caroline, a carer who has lots of experience in both carers' and disabled people's organisations, says it is important to be absolutely frank.

Caroline

'Make sure they know what you *can't* do – not what you can. The definition of something you can't do is simple. If you cannot do it every day as often as you want without help, however small that help might be, then you cannot do it. Don't put on a brave face. In my experience you cannot be brave *and* get what you want.'

Needs could be written down and a copy given to the interviewer. Consider every aspect of living – getting up, washing, going to the toilet and bathing, dressing, cleaning, getting around the house, cooking, laundry, shopping, paying bills and completing forms, going out, taking holidays, companionship and so on. Make sure that every difficulty is included, however trivial it may seem. The assessment is your relative's chance to have their say about what help they feel they need.

Local authorities can directly provide services themselves or make arrangements for private or voluntary sector organisations to provide care on their behalf. If a local authority is arranging or providing services, it will usually then carry out a financial assessment to find out how much the person should contribute towards the cost of those services. This financial assessment should take place separately from the assessment of needs, although in practice this may be difficult to distinguish.

After the assessment, the interviewer should record the individual's needs in writing and give them a copy. Social services will then specify which services they can offer to meet those needs and at what cost. This will be called a 'care package' or a 'care plan'. There is a right of appeal – both about the type of care being offered and about the cost – and in most cases the individual can turn down any services they do not want.

Penny

'I found that I lived in a fairly open-minded authority – they included independent living in their provision. At that time social services could provide 40 hours a week of help from personal (care) assistants. And I got a car through Motability.'

The assessment should also identify unmet needs – needs that exist but which the local authority cannot meet.

The individual may not get or be entitled to all the services they want. In this case, ask what the local authority's assessment criteria are. All local authorities have thresholds or other criteria that they use to decide who should receive a certain service and who should not, although some may deny this. Criteria often change in April – the beginning of a new financial year.

If your relative does not get what they need, it is worth seeking assistance from a law centre, advice agency or the disability organisation RADAR (address on page 149). Remember to keep copies of all letters you send and make a note of every phone call, including the name of the person you spoke to.

You have a right to complain to the council which must have a formal complaints procedure which is explained to you. A contact number within the authority should be given. Cases of maladministration (such as neglect, unjustifiable delay, unfair discrimination or failure to have the proper procedures or to abide by them) can be taken to the Local Government Ombudsman and/or to the Local Government Monitoring Officer (a senior local authority official). The local authority will provide names and addresses for both of these. Ultimately, an appeal can be made to the Secretary of State for Health.

If the local authority's action is unlawful, it may be possible, as a last resort, to sue them for breach of statutory duty but this is hard to prove. It is worth bringing any action of the local authority that might be unlawful to the attention of the Monitoring Officer, who is there to see that the authority acts within the law. An alternative is to ask the High Court for a judicial review if the local authority has behaved illegally, irrationally or failed to follow the correct procedures. If you are considering this, talk first to someone at a law centre, advice bureau or specialist disability organisation, and certainly to your MP.

Direct payments

Under the *Community Care (Direct Payments) Act 1996*, local authorities can, instead of providing services themselves, pay money directly to the individual so that they can buy the services they need. Or the person can opt for a mix of services and direct payments.

A direct payment is not extra income – it must be used to arrange services to meet assessed community care needs, including short periods of respite care. But it is up to the recipient to decide how their needs are met, by whom and when. Direct payments are not taxed or taken into account when assessing income for social security benefits.

The advantages of direct payments are obvious. Someone needing help getting out of bed in the morning, for example, may find that the home care assistant employed by the local authority cannot come at the time they want. With direct payments, however, they can arrange for someone else to come at whatever times they want. This can be done either by employing care staff directly or by using a home care agency of the person's choice. The recipient of the direct payment can specify what they want done, how and when, with direct reporting to the recipient.

New guidance makes it mandatory for local authorities to offer direct payments. The local authority should offer direct payments to anybody who meets the national eligibility criteria and who they are satisfied is able and willing to manage them, with – and this is an important point for carers – help if necessary. The criteria for receiving direct payments mainly limit access by people with mental health problems, on probation or with a drug addiction. Most people with arthritis should be eligible to receive them.

Arranging care through direct payments may sound daunting but why shouldn't people with care needs do what millions of working people do already – arrange domestic help with a third party? The local authority should have a support service that can answer queries, and invaluable information and advice can be obtained from the National Centre for Independent Living (NCIL) which publishes a leaflet called *The Art of Persuasion* about setting up a support scheme locally. Direct payments put the recipient in control – not the local authority and not the carer – and that is what most people with arthritis want.

Penny

'We've a direct payments users' group, which is a source of mutual support and advice, and the local authority has an independent living co-ordinator who works with us. I employ three PAs, and the paperwork – National Insurance, tax, public liability insurance – takes just an hour a week. Less now that I have a computer package to help.'

In England and Wales local authorities can also give carers direct payments (see page 75). To receive a direct payment, just as with a service, you must be assessed as providing regular and substantial care for someone who might need a community care service.

Independent Living (1993) Fund

People receiving substantial help from their local authority may have access to the Independent Living (1993) Fund. This is a trust financed by the government but administered by seven independent trustees to provide cash payments to severely disabled people under the age of 66. It helps people to live at home rather than in residential care by helping them to meet the additional costs of their domestic or personal care.

The Fund works in partnership with local authorities to enable jointly financed packages of care to be arranged. At the time of writing (2003), if a local authority is providing services and/or direct payments to a minimum value of £200 net a week, the Fund can consider making cash payments of up to £395 a week directly to the disabled person. This must be used to employ people as care assistants. It is not for aids or adaptations, bills or other costs. The primary responsibility for care needs remains with the local authority.

Access to the Independent Living (1993) Fund doesn't depend on a person's National Insurance contributions although account will be taken of their income. It is not available to anyone who has savings of more than £18,500.

For more information

𝒊 Age Concern Factsheets (see page 157 for details of how to obtain factsheets):

24 *Direct Payments from Social Services*

32 *Disability and Ageing: Your Rights to Social Services*

41 *Local Authority Assessment for Community Care Services.*

𝒊 For more information on independent living, contact the **National Centre for Independent Living** (address on page 147), which can direct you to your local centre. It can also provide further information on direct payments.

𝒊 Arthritis Care booklet *Reaching Independence: A Guide to Living at Home for People with Arthritis* (address on page 141).

𝒊 Contact the **Independent Living Fund** (address on page 146).

Family

If you are caring for a relative, do not feel obliged to take all responsibility for caring on yourself. Other members of the family can lend a hand, even if you are the closest relative. Think broadly. Even people who live a long way away can provide occasional help – a break away for you or the person for whom you are caring, for example.

Together, make a list of all the tasks that need attention and of everyone who can help. The list you both made for a social services assessment would be a good start but it will be useful to go into even more detail. It's easier to encourage people to help when the tasks are small – they can see that they will be able to cope.

To build support for the arrangements, the best bet is to try to get people to volunteer for particular tasks. People with cars can help with shopping or going out. Younger members of the family can pop in on the way from school or college. Working people might prefer to help financially rather than practically, by paying for a particular service or household aid. They will feel much more comfortable about doing this if they can see that everyone else is doing their bit. Whatever is going to be done, encourage the family member to discuss it with their relative who will be on the receiving end.

Voluntary organisations

The two obvious places you can turn to are carers' organisations and organisations for people with arthritis. Arthritis Care is the UK's leading voluntary organisation for people with arthritis, and can supply the names and addresses of the organisations that deal with specific types of arthritis. The leading carers' organisation is Carers UK, which has a UK-wide network of offices, branches and members. These provide information, advice and support as well as a voice for carers.

Caroline

'It was the counsellor I saw when I was depressed who first pointed out that I was a full-time carer as well as a full-time worker. It was the first time I'd heard the word. She suggested I go to a meeting with other carers, and I became quite involved. It helped put my own problems in perspective, and at various times I think we all broke down in front of each other. That gave us strength. After my husband Jeff died, I took up campaigning for carers with the local authority and also nationally. Finding a network of people is very important. I didn't realise at first just how important. I don't know if I would have got by without that bedrock, and I also made some strong friendships which I still maintain.'

There are also many local carers' groups or there may be a carers' centre in the area funded by a charity such as The Princess Royal Trust for Carers (address on page 148) or by the local health or social services. Some day centres or family doctor practices have carers' groups attached to them too. Look up 'carer' in the local phone book, the Internet or ask at the local library, Citizens Advice or social services office.

For more *i*nformation

i Contact the various organisations mentioned for further information on how they can help. Their addresses are in the 'Useful addresses' section at the back of this book.

Paid care assistants

There are private agencies that can provide qualified nurses or care assistants. Some helpers will not undertake more than light household duties. Agencies that provide nurses or care workers who carry out personal care tasks are going to have to be registered with the National Care Standards Commission (which will become the Commission for Social Care Inspection in 2004) and comply with minimum standards. These standards will include written contracts with users.

Each agency has its own system for placing staff and charges and styles of service vary considerably. The advantages of an agency are that it should provide fully refereed staff with back-up in the event of sickness. It will also deal with tax and National Insurance. But it will probably be more expensive than recruiting someone yourself.

The charity Counsel and Care (address on page 144) has a database of home care agencies. The UK Home Care Association (UKHCA) is a professional body for agencies providing care at home (address on page 150). It can tell you of any members in your area and also produces a free leaflet called *Choosing Care in Your Home*. Alternatively, you can look under 'Nurses' Agencies and Care Agencies' in *Yellow Pages*.

Bringing a professional into a personal relationship can sometimes have its problems, as Diane found. She has had arthritis since she was 18 months old, and one of her carers is her mother.

Diane

'It's difficult to get the balance. She's my mother but I'm an adult. With a paid carer you can state what you want and how you want it done. You can't do that with your mum.

'It was difficult when I first employed a personal assistant. My mum felt she was being pushed out. But we're open and we talk about things. Although parents can be over-protective of disabled children, my mum respects me as a person with my own opinions. I involved her in the interviewing for my personal assistant, which I think helped. It's meant that we've both got time and space away from each other. Now, I'm very close to my mum. We have a nice relationship.'

To find someone yourself, you can advertise in the local paper or JobCentre. The national magazines *The Lady* and *Choice* are also widely used for this sort of advertising. If you do advertise, it is advisable to use a box number and to take up references. Think carefully about what you actually need. Is it a qualified nurse or just someone who'll be there when needed? Penny has had about seven personal assistants (PAs) over the years.

> ### *Penny*
>
> 'Finding the right PA is very important; they need to understand the distinction between a PA and a carer. The main thing is to be clear about what you want. You need to find the right place to advertise for a PA or go to an agency. I use *The Big Issue* and the local paper.
>
> 'I chat to people for quite a long time and I'm fairly upfront about what I want. Being clear about what is needed is vital and that's why I provide a list of exactly what needs to be done. I want to put off people who aren't suitable and I interview only the two or three who seem most appropriate. For me, feeling they'll fit into my life is more important than experience. I have interviewed people who have no experience and are worried about that. I'm not. If someone hasn't done it before, they'll do it my way. Our independent living group has designed an application form that I use. Most local schemes will have one. Timing is important, too. The summer is never very good for recruiting.
>
> 'If you are worried about interviewing prospective PAs, get a friend or an advocate or someone from your local independent living group to help. It's not as hard as you might think.'

If you do the recruiting yourself, check out the references and be prepared to take on the responsibilities of an employer – including a contract of terms and conditions, Statutory Sick Pay, National Insurance contributions, Income Tax and insurance. Needless to say, discuss it all with the person who will be receiving the care, regardless of who is actually doing the hiring.

For more *i*nformation

ⓘ For information about hiring someone yourself, get the *Personal Assistants Employer's Handbook*, published by the West of England Centre for Inclusive Living (address on page 150).

ⓘ **The National Centre for Independent Living** (address on page 147) can also provide further information on employing personal assistants.

5 Planning for change

It is all very well reading about the things discussed in this book but at some point you and the person you are caring for will have to act on some of them. You will certainly have to plan for them. But how do you do that?

It is easy to say that it's the decision of the person with arthritis but it's never as simple as that. Making a decision is difficult. And once it's made, expressing it can be even harder. This chapter looks at how you can talk together to try to ensure that, as far as possible, what happens to them is what the person with arthritis wants.

Jack

'It's easy to say "Talk about it" but you have to make sure that it actually happens and that you talk properly. Turn off the telly, turn off the radio and sit down together.'

You will need to be open minded. This may mean challenging some of your own views about the right and wrong way to live. Try asking questions rather than giving what you think are the answers. When discussing the way forward for you both, it is important that each of you feels able to be honest about what you want. Although the person you are caring for should make decisions about their life, your life is equally important and there should be room for give and take on both sides.

Important discussions such as these can be exhausting, so aim to take a break after an hour and a half. And don't aim to resolve everything in one session. You may find that you will both want to mull over what each other has said and come back to the subject some days later.

Three key questions

Few problems are straightforward and, when it comes to caring, it is probably fair to say that none of them is. Everything is related to something else, and it can be difficult to know where to start talking. But there are three key questions to keep in your mind, however complicated the discussion gets:

- Where is the person with arthritis now? (the current situation)
- Where do they want to be? (the preferred situation)
- How do they get there? (the route)

The attitudes with which you embark on these discussions will make a big difference to how you both feel about them and their outcomes. You will need to show the person you are caring for and their views:

- **respect** – which involves accepting their concerns, however unfounded they may seem, giving them your full attention, time and effort, and letting them know that you believe they are capable of making their own decisions;
- **empathy** – trying to understand how they feel, not deciding how you think they ought to feel or projecting onto them how you might feel in a similar situation; and
- **genuineness** – meaning what you say and saying what you mean in a tactful but not a defensive, emotional or manipulative way.

How to listen effectively

Body language does make a difference. Remember SOLER:

S face the other person **S**quarely;

O sit **O**penly without crossed arms and legs;

L **L**ean towards the other attentively;

E maintain **E**ye contact;

R be **R**elaxed.

All this can help you to encourage the person you are caring for to speak frankly. You will certainly want to think about the ways of listening that promote communication:

- **active** – listening, nodding and giving verbal encouragement to go on;
- **attentive** – not interrupting but maintaining encouraging eye contact;
- **reflecting** – bouncing back something that has been said to encourage more and to check that you have understood; and
- **paraphrasing** – summarising what has just been said, to make sure that you really understand what is being said and how the person feels about it.

You will want to ask questions. Indeed, you will need to ask questions. But ask only one at a time. Multiple questions – Have you X; what about Y; do you want Z? – are confusing. And avoid asking leading questions of the variety 'Wouldn't it be great if you did this?'

Closed questions (ones to which the answer is 'Yes' or 'No') are best to ascertain matters of fact. Open questions (such as 'What do you think about that?') are better for drawing out feelings. Try to be gently probing rather than blunt. 'Why did you do that?' can sound threatening and prompt a defensive response. 'How did you feel about what happened?' is much warmer.

The person you are talking to will have their own prejudices just like everyone else, and these may be getting in the way of their making a decision. For example, misconceptions about what retirement housing actually is might prevent its being considered. Sometimes ignorance may be the problem. For example, not claiming a benefit because the person doesn't know it exists. You need to address these by challenging – again gently. 'What do you think stops you from doing Z?' or 'What do you think about Y?'

Even in the example of the unclaimed benefit, a tentative approach is best. Don't say 'You should claim Housing Benefit'. Letting the person with arthritis make the decision for themselves isn't just about showing respect, it's practical from your point of view too. The person will be much more committed to the idea if they come to it themselves.

Setting goals

What we want is rarely as simple as deciding whether to have tea or coffee with our breakfast. We normally work within a hazy framework of vague aspirations and unstated intentions. Distilling these into clear goals will help you both a lot. It's easy to say what these goals might be in general terms – staying in my own home, reducing my medication, taking more exercise – but clear goals may only emerge after going around a lot of conversational houses.

Goals should be:

- **Specific** Words such as 'better' aren't helpful. If the goal is to lose weight, how much weight? This makes it far easier to know whether (or when) the goal has been achieved.
- **Attainable** Achievable short-term targets are better than pie-in-the-sky long-term ideals. To have more money might be a desirable goal but, if someone is claiming all the benefits they are entitled to and cannot work, it may not be achievable. Breaking up a major task into small, attainable chunks can really help here.
- **Relevant** The goal has to be something the person wants to achieve – not a goal imposed from outside – and one that really will take them closer to where they want to be.

List all the possible goals and assess each on its merits as seen by the person with arthritis before choosing one or two to focus on.

Taking action

Question three – how to get there? – is the tough one but you don't need to know the answers. You just need to know the questions. Between you, think of all the possible ways of achieving the goal, however ridiculous they may seem. This is sometimes called brainstorming. You'll probably have a laugh doing it and come up with a longish list for even the most impossible-seeming idea. Assess all the options. If there truly isn't a route to the desired goal, you might have to reconsider question two – where does the person want to be? The conversation may go back and forth here.

Once a route is identified, you might want to think about an action plan. What needs to be done and in what order? By whom? By when? What information do you need? What problems might arise and how might they be overcome?

The three-question approach is flexible and will work with virtually any situation, from a simple one such as whether to buy a back-support cushion to a complex one such as where to live. Sometimes it will work very informally; on other occasions it might make sense to write down your lists of ideas and actions. The approach works on a number of levels. On the way to one major goal – living independently in my own home – there may be a number of intermediate goals, such as getting an assessment, claiming all my benefits, getting the bathroom altered and so on. It can help whenever there is difference between what is and what is desired.

Asking the three key questions is not original. If you go for counselling – and many people with arthritis and those caring for them benefit from it – you will probably find that they use a similar approach. And don't be surprised if you find the person you are caring for trying it out on you.

> ### Fiona
>
> 'I didn't just come straight out and tell my mother I was getting a professional carer. I talked to her about the problems my needs were causing for her in running her own life. Her relationship with my dad, her relationship with my sister who lives quite a long way away, the fact that her career was on hold – all these came up when we were talking. It wasn't easy at first. She did her usual routine – knocking back her tea saying "Well, I must get on". I moved the conversation on myself I suppose by taking her hand and telling her how much I valued what she did. That got her talking to me seriously. That and the fact that I stuck my wheelchair between her and the kitchen door!'

For more *i*nformation

i The **British Association for Counselling and Psychotherapy** (address on page 142) can supply a list of counsellors in your area.

6 What do you need to think about?

The previous chapter considered how you and the person you are caring for might approach problem solving. This chapter looks at some of the specific problems you might need to solve, and offers some of the information and advice that might help you to do that.

Prakash

'It sounds such a simple thing but the turning point was when we just sat down and made a list. We realised that we needed to think about the problems or difficulties that the arthritis had created. Then we could find out the necessary information and work out how to solve them – with help if we needed it.'

Long-term medical prognosis

To make the best caring choices, it is important to get a good idea of how the arthritis is going to develop. A social services assessment will help but ideally you should both discuss the prognosis with the GP or consultant. Doctors can sometimes feel uncomfortable about being put on the spot like this but, if you explain why you are asking, most will try to be helpful. Make sure that the people you are dealing with, particularly social services, know the prognosis. Having the right aids and adaptations in place promptly can reduce joint damage and subsequent loss of mobility.

Rheumatoid arthritis varies considerably in severity. Perhaps a third of people who develop rheumatoid arthritis will only ever have very mild disease. The majority will have periods of remission but also more serious pain, swelling and flares throughout their lives. Possibly 5 per cent develop severe disease with extensive disability but even in this group many people continue to live independently. Initially it may be difficult to tell which category an individual will be in but improved testing is making this easier.

In most cases osteoarthritis will get worse with time but it is generally steady, which makes planning a little easier.

Dealing with crises

In older people, arthritis can come on very suddenly, particularly rheumatoid arthritis. It can be triggered by a crisis. Brenda's came on after a heart operation.

Brenda

'It started in Bognor on holiday. We'd been walking all day and at about midnight I just couldn't breathe. I was rushed into hospital. They did some tests and found I had a leaky heart valve that had to be replaced. I'd always had high blood pressure and high cholesterol. I think the heart problem triggered everything else. The body is like an old car, I suppose – once something goes, everything else starts to pack in.

'The arthritis came on when I was in rehabilitation after the heart operation but I couldn't understand it at first. It was far worse than any pain I'd had before and that includes the night I was rushed to hospital with my heart. One night I woke up and my wrist was aching. It quickly moved to my knee and then to my feet. Blood tests confirmed that I had rheumatoid arthritis. I think it was the shock of the operation or perhaps a reaction to one of the many antibiotics I had afterwards that triggered it.'

In the event of any sudden change in circumstances, including rapid onset of the disease, the local authority can provide emergency services (under section 47 of the *NHS and Community Care Act 1990*) before a full needs assessment has been made.

Falls are a particular risk for people with arthritis. They are more likely to happen and their impact can be more serious. (Some suggestions for reducing the risks are given on page 125.) In most cases, a person with arthritis who has a fall should have an X-ray to check that there is no damage. Even if nothing is broken, they are likely to stiffen up – which may increase care needs for a few days.

If the person is taken into hospital, make sure you know when they will be discharged. Hospitals should not discharge someone after a fall, for example, without ensuring that any care needs at home will be met. Don't rush into making changes in care or domestic arrangements after a fall but, equally, don't assume that its effects will disappear with the bruises. Confidence is likely to be affected – for many people, a fall becomes symbolic of losing control of one's life. Time and encouragement are the best you can give in these circumstances.

For more *i*nformation

i Age Concern Factsheet 37 *Hospital Discharge Arrangements* (see page 157 for details of how to obtain factsheets).

Money

Money management

Disability can be expensive. Housing, transport and day-to-day household expenses often cost more when you have arthritis. Many of these costs are reflected in the costs of caring. Even if the person is living independently or in a care home, you will still probably incur additional transport costs from more frequent visits, higher telephone bills and the cost of any fees, aids or alterations to which you contribute. If someone is living in your home, you will need to think about additional food, heating, transport, living aids and adaptations to your home.

Extra costs of living with arthritis include:

- additional heating and hot water;
- personal assistance;
- domestic help;
- gardening and household maintenance;
- home adaptations;
- special equipment;
- mobility – car adaptations and taxi fares;
- special diets;
- prescription and non-prescription drugs; and
- non-NHS treatment, such as complementary therapies.

It is unlikely that you will need to take over formal responsibility for the finances of someone whose only impairment is arthritis but it is important that both of you know exactly what your income and expenses are. An open relationship about money and clear, transparent practices are important. Most family rows are over money, and a caring relationship might complicate matters still further.

If money is a problem for you, don't be embarrassed about seeking help. Many local authorities have a specialist money advice worker. The local Citizens Advice can also be very helpful. A money adviser will take you through your finances systematically and show you how to maximise income and minimise expenditure. It really can work – especially when you feel that you just cannot make ends meet.

State benefits

This section looks at the benefits available to you both. Neither you nor the person you are caring for should have any qualms about claiming these benefits. Millions of pounds in benefits go unclaimed every week by those entitled to them, particularly among older people.

The information here is as accurate as possible but benefits, rates and the regulations governing them do change. The Benefits Enquiry Line for people with disabilities on 0800 88 22 00, will give you confidential information on the current position. Your local Citizens Advice may have a benefits adviser who can advise you both about the benefits to which you are entitled, or try the local welfare rights group or local Age Concern.

Benefits that depend on the claimant having paid sufficient National Insurance contributions are known as *contributory*. Those that depend on how much money or savings the person has are known as *income related* or *means tested*. Some benefits are taxable although, of course, you will only have to pay tax on them if your total taxable income – including these benefits – exceeds your tax allowance.

This section is divided into four parts:

- benefits for the person with arthritis;
- benefits for carers;
- benefits for people with a State Pension; and
- benefits for people on low incomes.

Benefits for the person with arthritis

There are many benefits that can be claimed by an ill or disabled person. The local social security or Pension Service office will have leaflets and application forms, which will give full details. There is only room in this book to consider some of the main ones that may be relevant to you and the person you are caring for.

Attendance Allowance

Attendance Allowance is a tax-free, non-contributory, non-means-tested benefit for people aged 65 and over who need help with personal care or need someone to watch over them because of physical or mental illness or disability. These needs must normally have existed for at least six months. The allowance does not have to be used to pay for care, but the local authority can take it into account when assessing whether and how much a person should pay for any social services they receive.

There is a higher and a lower rate. The *lower rate* is paid if the person needs frequent help throughout the day or at least twice at night. The *higher rate* is paid if the person needs such help during the day *and* at night.

Disability Living Allowance

Like Attendance Allowance, this is a tax-free, non-contributory, non-means-tested benefit. The person will have become disabled and made a claim before the age of 65 because they need help with personal care or getting around, or both. Normally, these needs must have existed for three months and be expected to continue for at least another six months. There are two components: the care component and the mobility component.

The **care component** is for people needing personal care (such as help with washing, dressing or cooking). It is paid at three rates, according to the amount of care required:

- the *higher rate* if help is needed both day and night;
- the *middle rate* if help is needed day or night; or
- the *lower rate* if some help is needed during some of the day.

Payment of the benefit may stop if the claimant moves into a care home.

The **mobility component** is for people who need help getting around. This is paid at two rates: higher and lower.

The *higher rate* is paid to a number of categories of people. The relevant category for someone with arthritis is that of people who cannot walk at all or are virtually unable to walk. People receiving this higher rate may be exempt from road tax; they can also apply to the local authority for a Blue Badge (previously called an Orange Badge) and they may be able to get a car or electric wheelchair under the Motability scheme (see address on page 147).

The *lower rate* is payable if a claimant can walk but is unable to do so out of doors unless someone is with them.

The mobility component of Disability Living Allowance is not affected by moving into a care home.

To claim, the person completes form DLA 1, which includes a section for the claimant's own assessment of how their illness or disability affects them. The form is quite long but do not be put off by this. A medical examination will not normally be necessary. A local advice agency may be able to help with the form or you can ring the Benefits Enquiry Line for advice on 0800 88 22 00. If it is difficult for the claimant to get out, the local social security office may be able to arrange for a visiting officer to call to help with the form.

Payment of Disability Living Allowance may be combined with other benefits so that they are all paid together.

Severe disability premium

This may be payable to a disabled person who lives alone and receives Attendance Allowance or the middle or higher level of the care component of the Disability Living Allowance and no one is receiving Carer's Allowance (previously called Invalid Care Allowance) for looking after them. It may also be payable to someone living with a partner who also receives Attendance Allowance. The rules are complicated, so it is best to seek advice before claiming this premium.

Under Pension Credit, introduced in October 2003, the guarantee credit replaced Income Support (also known as Minimum Income Guarantee) for people aged 60 and over. There are additional amounts for severely disabled people and carers, which are the same as the current severe disability and carer premiums.

Statutory Sick Pay

An employee who is under 65 and earning at least a certain amount (£77 a week in 2003), and who has to take time off sick with arthritis will probably be entitled to Statutory Sick Pay (SSP), just like any other member of staff. It is paid, by the employer, for up to 28 weeks.

Incapacity Benefit

Incapacity Benefit is for people under State Pension age who cannot work because of illness or disability. It cannot be claimed by anyone who was over the State Pension age when their illness began. It is paid at three rates:

- at the *short-term lower rate* for the first 28 weeks of illness, to people who are self-employed, unemployed, non-employed or employed but not eligible for Statutory Sick Pay;
- at the *short-term higher rate* from week 29 to week 52 of their illness to all the above plus employees who have received Statutory Sick Pay; or
- at the *long-term rate* to all the above from week 53 of their illness.

An important exception here concerns people receiving Disability Living Allowance (discussed above). People claiming the care component of Disability Living Allowance at the highest rate are entitled to the long-term rate of Incapacity Benefit from week 29 of their illness rather than from week 53. This also applies to people who are terminally ill.

For the first 28 weeks, a doctor's certificate of inability to work should be sufficient. After that, most people will have to undertake a 'personal capability assessment'. This will involve a questionnaire and, in some cases, a medical examination.

Under the 'permitted work rules' people receiving Incapacity Benefit can work for up to 16 hours a week, on average, and earn up to no more than a set limit a week for 26 weeks. In some cases this can be extended by a further 26 weeks if the adviser at the Jobcentre Plus office agrees.

Occupational or personal pensions of more than a set amount (£85 a week in 2003) will normally reduce the amount of benefit – for every £1 of pension more than £85, 50 pence of benefit will be lost. This rule does not apply, however, to anyone receiving Incapacity benefit before April 2001 nor to new claimants in receipt of the highest rate of the care component of Disability Living Allowance.

The long-term rate of Incapacity Benefit cannot be paid after State Pension age. So once someone reaches pension age (currently 60 for women, 65 for men), they should draw the State Pension.

Working Tax Credit

Working Tax Credit was introduced in April 2003. It replaced the Disabled Person's Tax Credit (and Working Families' Tax Credit). It is administered by the Inland Revenue and the assessment of income and savings is different to the rules for social security benefits.

People with a disability that puts them at a disadvantage in the job market and are receiving certain benefits, such as Disability Living Allowance or Attendance Allowance, and are working at least 16 hours per week may get the tax credit from the Inland Revenue. Whether a person qualifies and, if so, the level of the credit depends on their circumstances, their income (including that of their partner if they have one) and whether they qualify for the disability or the 50 plus elements.

Many working people with arthritis will be eligible. For more information ring the Tax Credits Helpline on 0845 300 3900 or look at the website at www.inlandrevenue.gov.uk/taxcredits

Benefits for carers

Carer's Allowance

This is a non-contributory, non-means-tested, taxable, weekly benefit for people of working age who are giving 'regular and substantial' care at least 35 hours a week to a severely disabled person who is receiving Attendance Allowance or Disability Living Allowance at the highest or middle rate of the care component. Until April 2003 it was called Invalid Care Allowance. The person being cared for does not have to be a relative and may live separately or with you.

There is now no upper age limit for claiming Carer's Allowance, but if you are receiving a State Pension or another benefit you may not receive the allowance on top of this.

Carer's Allowance cannot be claimed by someone who is earning more than a set amount (£77 a week in 2003). If another social security benefit such as the State Pension, Widow's Pension or

Incapacity Benefit is being claimed and the amount received is less than the Carer's Allowance, the difference can be made up to the weekly rate for that allowance. If another benefit is being claimed and the amount received is higher than the Carer's Allowance, that allowance is not paid.

If you have a low income it may still be worth claiming, however, even though it may not be paid in addition to your current benefit or pension. Although Carer's Allowance is counted as income if you claim Income Support, Pension Credit, Housing Benefit or Council Tax Benefit, people entitled to Carer's Allowance may be able to get higher rates of these benefits because of the 'carer premium' (carer addition in Pension Credit).

In some situations the person you care for could lose money if you start to receive Carer's Allowance. This will apply if they receive the severe disability premium (see page 109) as part of their Income Support, Housing Benefit or Council Tax Benefit, or the severe disability addition in Pension Credit.

A claim can be backdated for up to three months. Don't delay making a claim for Carer's Allowance because you are waiting to hear if the person you care for is eligible for Attendance Allowance or Disability Living Allowance: get claim pack DS 700 from your local social security office or by ringing the Benefit Enquiry Line on Freephone 0800 88 22 00.

Home Responsibilities Protection

If you are looking after a disabled person and cannot work or do not pay enough National Insurance contributions to count for State Pension purposes, you may be entitled to Home Responsibilities Protection (HRP). This protects your State Pension. HRP reduces the number of qualifying years needed for a Basic State Pension. The minimum number of years to which it can be reduced is 20.

If you get Carer's Allowance you will normally be getting National Insurance credits towards your pension so you will not need HRP. If not, ask for claim form CF 411 from the Jobcentre Plus office.

Benefits for people with a State Pension

Benefits that can be claimed by someone already receiving a State Pension include Attendance Allowance, Christmas Bonus, Council Tax Benefit, Disability Living Allowance, Housing Benefit, Income Support, help with NHS costs, Over-80s Pension Category D, Pension Credit, War Disablement Pension, War Pensioner's Mobility Supplement, War Widow's Pension, Widow's Pension and Winter Fuel Payments. Contact a local advice agency for more information.

Benefits for people on low incomes

The benefits that can be claimed by people on low incomes include Council Tax Benefit, Housing Benefit, Income Support, Pension Credit, Jobseeker's Allowance and help with NHS costs.

Depending on your exact circumstances, you might want to explore your own entitlement and that of the person for whom you are caring to the following:

Income Support This is a benefit which helps with weekly basic living expenses by topping up income to a level set by the Government. It is also a passport to other benefits, such as community care grants from the Social Fund, Cold Weather Payments, Housing Benefit, and free NHS dental treatment for example.

Pension Credit In October 2003 the guarantee credit replaced Income Support for people aged 60 and over. The savings credit provides additional money to people aged 65 and over who have income over a certain level.

Housing Benefit and Council Tax Benefit These are payable by the local authority to people on low incomes who need help to pay their rent or Council Tax.

Tips on claiming benefits

- If in doubt, claim. Citizens Advice locally or the Carers UK CarersLine (see page 143) can do a benefits check for you to make sure you are not overlooking anything.

■ Be honest about what you are unable to do. Put simply, if you cannot do something as often as you want, you *cannot* do it even if you can do it occasionally or only need a little help.

■ With benefits that include premiums, make sure that you are getting all you are entitled to.

■ If you are going to claim a disability benefit, you may wish to get information first from a local disability group or call Arthritis Care's helpline (see page 141). Talk to them again if you are turned down and plan to appeal.

For more *i*nformation

i Your Rights: *A Guide to Money Benefits for Older People*, published annually by Age Concern Books (see page 156).

i *Benefits for Beginners*, a booklet from Arthritis Care (see address on page 141).

i Age Concern has a number of factsheets that may be of help (see page 157 for details of how to obtain factsheets):

17 *Housing Benefit and Council Tax Benefit*

18 *A Brief Guide to Money Benefits*

25 *Income Support*

34 *Attendance Allowance and Disability Living Allowance*

48 *Pension Credit*

49 *Help from the Social Fund.*

Pensions

You are entitled to a State Pension when you reach State Pension age – currently 60 for a woman, 65 for a man – if you have paid or been credited with enough National Insurance (NI) contributions. The amount you receive is not affected by your income and savings but it is taxable.

The Basic State Pension is the same for men, for women who have paid their own standard-rate NI contributions and for widows who claim on their deceased husband's contributions. Married women who are not entitled on the basis of their own NI contributions may receive a pension on the basis of their husband's. A man who became a widower before the age of 65 who is not entitled to a full Basic Pension can have his wife's contributions taken into account to give him a higher pension.

You may also receive some Graduated Pension (officially called Graduated Retirement Benefit) if you paid employee National Insurance contributions between 1961 and 1975 and/or some Additional Pension built up under the State Earnings-Related Pension Scheme (SERPS) between 1978 and 2002 (or under the State Second Pension since April 2002).

You can increase your State Pension if you put off receiving it (called 'deferring' it) for up to five years after State Pension age and do not claim certain other benefits. If you defer drawing your pension, your Additional and Graduated Pensions will be increased in the same way as the Basic Pension. (See social security guide NP 46 for more information about deferring pensions.)

People receiving the State Pension can claim other benefits, including Pension Credit. Everyone over 60 is entitled to free NHS prescriptions and may get help with other health costs.

Men and women widowed before State Pension age may be entitled to bereavement benefits. They may be entitled to the Bereavement Payment and the Bereavement Allowance, depending on their late spouse's NI contribution record. People widowed after pension age may be entitled to claim a State Pension based on their late spouse's contributions.

You and/or the person you care for may be entitled to an occupational or personal pension. If you have paid into one, your employer or scheme provider should provide you with the relevant information. Seek advice if you are dissatisfied or concerned. If necessary, you can contact the Pensions Advisory Service (OPAS) at the address on page 148 or Citizens Advice.

For more *i*nformation

ⓘ Age Concern Factsheet 19 *The State Pension* (see page 157 for details of how to obtain factsheets).

ⓘ The Department for Work and Pensions produces a number of leaflets about State and other pensions – these can be obtained from the **Pensions Info-Line** on 0845 731 3233 or the website at www.dwp.gov.uk

ⓘ Contact the **Pensions Advisory Service** at the address on page 148.

Insurance

Check your entitlement to help under any insurance policies you or the person you are caring for might have. If you have private medical insurance, don't assume that you will be covered. Insurance companies don't like paying out, and when you are talking about a long-term condition such as arthritis they are very reluctant. Check the small print.

The Disability Discrimination Act 1995 makes it unlawful to discriminate against disabled people in connection with the provision of goods, facilities and services and this applies to insurance policies. However, insurance companies may be able to differentiate their policies for a person with disabilities (including arthritis) provided that the differentiation is based on information that is relevant to the assessment of risk being insured *and* the information on which this judgement is based is from a source on which it is reasonable to rely.

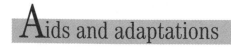

Aids and adaptations

Four main types of equipment are available:

- An item or gadget designed specifically for disabled people to overcome a particular difficulty (eg a wheelchair, bath board, raised toilet seat or orthopaedic footwear).
- Standard equipment with a particularly helpful feature that takes the physical effort out of the activity (eg an electric tin

opener, a food processor, a computer, Velcro fastenings or power steering on a car).

■ Standard equipment that has been adapted (eg a tap with a long handle, a comb with a long handle).

■ A 'custom made' item to suit a particular individual's need. These can be made at home, commercially or by the voluntary organisation REMAP.

Below are some examples of the types of aids that may be particularly useful for a person with arthritis:

■ People with weak or painful hands often prefer lightweight gadgets or appliances with larger, easy-to-grip controls or handles that require less force. Rubber knob turners can change fiddly controls into easy ones. A person with arthritis might also benefit from a gadget being secured in place so that one hand is not needed to hold or steady it – a slicing guide for bread, for example.

■ People using wheelchairs will need sufficient space for turning and transferring. They need appliances that are positioned so they can be operated within their reach from the chair and with sufficient knee room to get in close. Cooker controls must be at the front of the cooker, for example.

■ People who find it difficult to bend may need long-handled equipment – grabbers, reachers or pick-up sticks. Gadgets need to be positioned above waist height, including, for example, electric socket extenders. Raised seats may be helpful, but this need not mean buying new furniture – specially designed wooden blocks can do the job. The legs need to fit snugly into the raised blocks; simply resting them on a brick or something similar could be dangerous.

■ Most people with arthritis will want appliances that aren't tiring to use. This includes labour-saving devices such as washing machines, electric wheelchairs and food processors as well as smaller gadgets such as teapot pourers.

Clothing is a good example of how a little ingenuity goes a long way. With such a variety of fabrics, fastenings and styles to choose from, it is usually possible to find something that your relative will

feel good wearing and that they can actually get into. And think laterally. Why struggle with a tie when they can buy a clip-on? If they can't get a good loose fit in their size, buy larger sizes. Women could check out the larger, baggier sizes in the men's department.

Bigger buttons are easier than smaller ones. A big tab on a zip makes it easier to move – attaching a cord can also help. Velcro, with its hundreds of tiny fibre hooks, is easy to use. Accessible fastenings also help – front rather than back fastenings on bras, for example. Many popular items of clothing need no fastening at all, including jogging suits, tracksuits, shawls, wrap-around skirts and kimonos.

There are four ways to get hold of aids and equipment:

- through the occupational therapist from social services or the NHS;
- buying them privately, either new or second-hand;
- from charities or other organisations; or
- making them.

Getting equipment through social services or the health service

If your relative needs equipment to help them manage more easily around the home, contact the local authority social services department. You don't have to have a letter from their GP supporting their needs but this can sometimes speed up the process. Social services have responsibility for the aids needed for daily living, such as those for washing, eating, dressing or going to the toilet. They can also help with grab rails and disabled parking spaces. (See page 86 for how to approach social services.) Councils may provide free equipment but can make charges – practice varies. There will usually first be an assessment in the home by an occupational therapist (OT). Equipment is provided from a disability equipment store which in some areas may be run jointly with the local health trust or under contract by another organisation.

The NHS is responsible for the provision of 'personal mobility aids', such as wheelchairs, walking sticks and zimmer frames. The

NHS is not allowed to make charges for equipment but in some cases will ask for a returnable deposit for items.

Some of the medical items that will help someone with arthritis live at home can be prescribed by the GP – support bandages, for example – but most will require a referral. Physiotherapists can provide walking aids. Both physiotherapists and chiropodists may be able to help with footwear. A hospital foot specialist such as an orthotist or podiatrist certainly can. Community nurses can help with equipment for nursing someone at home, such as bedpans and hoists. Consultants may be able to help with special medical equipment.

Wheelchairs are usually provided through the NHS wheelchair service (ask the GP to refer you), which is able to provide a wide range of wheelchairs and cushions. Alternatively, they can give a voucher towards the person with arthritis buying one themselves.

It can be difficult to get equipment from social services or the health service. Sometimes there are strict eligibility criteria and there can also be long waiting times. Make sure that your GP is aware of any problems you have accessing statutory services, as a doctor or social worker's referral may get things moving.

Caroline

'Be honest with your GP about your problems. Don't kid yourself that you can cope. Ask politely for what you want. Don't wait to be asked or for it to be offered. Outline the difficulty clearly and say you want professional help to deal with it.

'I can't fault social services, but I knew the channels to go down. I made sure I knew everybody's name. They put in handrails, a bath unit, a special chair and offered a stairlift. Community care should be about outcomes not systems, and the outcomes should be based on the needs of the users. It must also be recognised that the needs of carers and of users are different. They will only come to understand this if we keep telling them.'

Buying equipment

With our growing older population, there is an expanding market for specialist aids and gadgets from jar openers and key turners to wheelchairs and stairlifts. You can find your local stores in the _Yellow Pages_ under 'Disabled Equipment', and some large chemist shops have a catalogue of equipment for people with disabilities. Do shop around, though. Many of the products and catalogues targeted specifically at disabled people are not good value for money. Some items are available more cheaply through mainstream outlets; others are simply not a lot of good. Discuss any possible purchase – particularly a larger one – with a health professional. Will it really help? It is possible to spend a lot of money on a product that is not really suitable.

A good retailer should allow you to try out a product either in the store or at home. Some stores may hire out equipment. Better still get independent or professional advice. At a Disabled Living Centre or Independent Living Centre you should be able to view and assess equipment with the benefit of an occupational therapist's advice and without the attentions of a shopkeeper. There are 49 Disabled Living Centres across the UK. For the address of the one nearest you, contact the Disabled Living Centres Council (see address on page 145) which also produces leaflets and reports about disability equipment.

The Disabled Living Foundation (DLF) also provides advice and information on disability equipment and assisted products. It has a national telephone enquiry service (see address on page 145) and produces factsheets and books on a variety of subjects, including choosing wheelchairs or other equipment. The DLF also has a factsheet listing journals that carry advertisements for second-hand equipment. Disabled Living Centres are also likely to have information about second-hand equipment available locally.

Equipment from charities

Some charities may also be able to help with the provision of equipment, either short term or long term. The British Red Cross, for example, lends basic items, including wheelchairs. Some charities may make a small charge.

Help paying for aids

Some financial help may be available for buying an item. Attendance Allowance and Disability Allowance are benefits which are intended to help disabled people meet the extra living costs (see pages 107–109). The government Social Fund can give community care grants to people on low incomes (see Age Concern Factsheet 49 *Help from the Social Fund*).

Some charities can also help with payment. The Association of Charity Officers and Charity Search (see addresses on pages 141 and 143) provide information on sources of funding for older people in need. The Disabled Living Foundation has a factsheet called *Raising Funds and Obtaining Equipment for Disabled People*. Most charities will want applications to be made through, or at least countersigned by, a social worker or health professional.

VAT is not charged on support aids and equipment provided that they are for the use of a disabled person. You will have to sign a declaration to that effect. Contact the local VAT office (see under 'Customs and Excise' in the phone book) and ask for VAT leaflet 701/7/94 *VAT Reliefs for People with Disabilities*.

Creative thinking

The more inventive prefer to make aids themselves. A visit to a Disabled Living Centre or disability aids shop can be a good source of inspiration.

In many cases, solving a problem may well be simpler than having an adaptation made to the house or even buying a gadget. Changing the way something is done may be all that is needed. If it is difficult to get in and out of the bath, a shower may be easier. If cooking is difficult or tiring, what about the possibilities offered by modern technology – the microwave, freezer and slow cooker, for example? If the difficulty is ironing, how about buying clothes that can be drip-dried?

It can be tough to change an activity that you have been doing in the same way for years – it can feel like a threat to your independence,

121

even your whole being. But if it results in an approach that is quicker, easier and less tiring, it must be worth considering.

For more *i*nformation

ⓘ Contact the **Disabled Living Foundation** at the address on page 145.

ⓘ Contact the **Disabled Living Centres Council** at the address on page 145.

ⓘ Age Concern Factsheet 42 *Disability Equipment and How to Get It* (see page 157 for details of how to obtain factsheets).

ⓘ Arthritis Care booklet *Reaching Independence* (address on page 141).

ⓘ *Your Home and Arthritis: An Information Booklet*, available free from the Arthritis Research Campaign (address on page 141).

Accommodation

Independent living

Independent living – that is, living in their own home – is likely to be the preferred option of most people with arthritis. Community care aims to facilitate this. Mobility problems are rarely insurmountable – a little ingenuity can go a long way – and social services are not the only body which may be able to help, as outlined in Chapter 4.

What, then, are the likely problems with independent living? Everyday tasks may be difficult: some may need to be done by someone else. The risk of accidents is real enough – probably far greater than the risk of crime. Loneliness can be overcome if family and friends live nearby and can visit regularly. By contrast, the advantages of not having to move and remaining independent in familiar surroundings are obvious.

Practical help in the home is discussed in Chapter 4; here we look at how the home can be adapted to make it more suitable. If major adaptations are being considered, information and advice on design issues and a database of architects, surveyors and similar professionals with experience of designing for disabled people are available from the Centre for Accessible Environments (address on page 143).

Alterations can be expensive, but you may be able to get a grant from the local authority towards the cost. Most grants are means-tested, so they will depend on the home owner's income and savings. There are two kinds of grants: mandatory grants are the grants the council has to pay if the work qualifies and a person's income and savings are low. With discretionary grants it is up to the council to decide whether to give them or not.

Disabled facilities grants can provide facilities and adaptations to help a disabled person to live as independently and in as much comfort as possible. The grants are mandatory in specific circumstances.

A grant must be given if a person is disabled and does not have access to their home and to the basic amenities within it, provided that they qualify on income grounds. The local authority also has to agree that the work is reasonable and that it is possible to carry it out.

Local authorities can also give discretionary assistance for adaptations or to help someone to move to alternative accommodation. It may be paid in addition or as an alternative to the grant.

In some areas there are home improvement agencies, often called 'Care and Repair' or 'Staying Put' projects, which help people needing to repair or adapt their homes. Ask the council if there is one or contact **'foundations'** at the address on page 146.

Grants for home insulation are made under the Warm Front Grant in England, the Home Energy Efficiency Scheme in Wales or the Warm Deal Scheme in Scotland. They are available to people aged 60 and over who receive certain State benefits.

■ *Never* **start the work before getting the local authority's approval to go ahead, or you will not be entitled to a grant.**

Brenda has rheumatoid arthritis and is cared for by her husband Tom.

Brenda

'We've had a lot of adaptations made to our house. The local authority have helped with some but not all and it's not been cheap. The alterations to the bathroom cost £3,400, and the firm didn't even redecorate.

'You need to be very careful. I saw one advert in a paper that said the company was recommended by Arthritis Care. I phoned the charity and they said it wasn't.'

Don't forget how much the local authority can help.

Tom

'We live in Lambeth, which must be one of the most criticised boroughs in the country but, once Brenda was registered disabled, we only had to wait four weeks before they painted a parking bay outside our house. They also fitted rails outside – we live on quite a steep hill – and smaller ones throughout the house. They also put an extra banister on the stairs. I knew all this was available because I used to do this sort of work myself when I worked at the local hospital.'

Brenda again

'We were lucky. Tom met an occupational therapist at an Arthritis Care meeting and she came round and had a look for us. One of the problems with rheumatologists is that they don't always tell the occupational therapist about you or you about them. Make sure you ask about them.'

For more *i*nformation

ⓘ For more information on independent living, contact the **National Centre for Independent Living** (address on page 147), which can direct you to your local centre.

ⓘ Age Concern Factsheet 13 *Older Home Owners: Financial Help with Repairs and Adaptations* (see page 157 for details of how to obtain factsheets).

ⓘ For more information about Warm Front Grants contact **EAGA (Energy Action Grants Agency)** at the address on page 145 or see Age Concern Factsheet 1 *Help with Heating.*

Reducing accidents

We all know the home can be a dangerous place but a little thought can make it much safer:

■ Falls are often caused by tripping, so grab rails are really useful.

■ Keep the floors in living areas free from clutter.

■ Trailing flexes can be tacked to the wall, or more sockets installed.

■ Go for simple floor-coverings. Fitted carpets are safer than slippery floors.

■ If there are mats, make sure they have non-slip strips fitted.

■ Worn stair carpet is particularly dangerous.

■ Reducing the need for stretching and reaching will also reduce the likelihood of accidents, so think about locations and accessibility of shelves and cupboards.

■ The impact of falls can be reduced by cushioning sharp edges and avoiding low level glass unless it is safety glass.

■ Non-safety glass can be coated with a shatterproof film to make it safer.

■ Plenty of lights with easy-to-use rocker or touch-sensitive switches will help.

■ Make sure that handles are easy to use and move readily. Long handles that are easier to turn are available for doors and taps.

Most accidents happen in the kitchen and bathroom. An accident in the kitchen is usually the result of knocking against something or trying to lift something too heavy; in the bathroom, from trying to manoeuvre in a small room with a slippery floor. To prevent accidents, think about how these rooms will be used. Work step by step through each process. Most problems can be solved. For example, instead of lifting a heavy pan of vegetables from the cooker to the sink, use a wire mesh basket of the type often used for chips to lift the vegetables out of the water. Make sure that all gas and electric appliances are checked regularly, and fit smoke alarms. Think about other gadgets that could reduce the risk of accidents – pill reminders, alarms, carbon monoxide detectors and so on.

For more *i*nformation

ⓘ For more advice on preventing accidents, contact the **Royal Society for the Prevention of Accidents** (RoSPA) at the address on page 149.

Retirement housing

Retirement housing, which is also known as sheltered accommodation, can be an option that gives the best of both worlds, providing much of the independence of living in one's own home but with a warden or manager nearby. The properties are usually purpose-built blocks of flats or bungalows designed for older people. Rented sheltered housing is generally provided by housing associations and local authorities. Private companies provide sheltered housing for sale, generally on a leasehold basis.

But there are some aspects to think carefully about. If the person with arthritis is considering buying, what exactly are they getting for their money? Some of these properties may not be particularly good value compared with others in the area, and whilst an older buyer will be thinking about present benefits rather than future investment, there is no point in paying over the odds. Whether renting or buying, it is important to know exactly what is being offered. Some include a shared lounge or laundry or other facilities, whereas others offer little more than an alarm system.

Whatever the case, how does the alarm work and when is the warden or manager on site?

Check out all the costs, particularly the service charges, very carefully as they may rise sharply. The local environment is also important, as it is whenever we move home. What facilities are nearby – shops, banks, post office, pharmacist/chemist shop, library, doctor's surgery, clubs, pubs, day centres, cinemas and so on? What transport is available? Is the area too hilly?

There are two codes of practice to look out for: the National House Building Council (NHBC) Sheltered Housing Code of Practice, which covers the building of properties; and the Association of Retirement Housing Managers Code of Practice, which covers the way in which they are managed. Under the NHBC code, purchasers should be given an information pack outlining exactly what, in terms of property and services, is being provided and by whom.

The local authority's housing department should be able to give information about retirement housing in the local area. The Elderly Accommodation Counsel (address on page 145) can also provide advice and lists of accommodation to rent or buy in all parts of the UK. Sheltered accommodation with extra arthritis care is provided by the Abbeyfield Society (national address on page 141), usually in larger houses converted into a number of bedsits.

For more *information*

❶ Age Concern Factsheets (see page 157 for details of how to obtain factsheets):

2 *Buying Retirement Housing*

8 *Looking For Rented Housing.*

Moving in with you

Moving someone with care needs into your home may seem like the obvious option but it is a big step for both of you. The privacy and independence of both parties is compromised and your relationship is complicated. It may be a very thorny issue when the person needing care is a relative. Some people have strong views about the role of family members, particularly that of women, and their obligations in caring for others in the family. You may hold some of these. So may the relative who needs care. Being open and talking it through is really the only way to address these issues.

Feeling that you don't want your relative to move in with you is nothing to be ashamed of. You get only one life and you have a right to yours, as have the other people who already live with you. Nobody should enter into this sort of arrangement just because they can't say 'No'. If the relationship is not strong enough for one of you to say 'I don't want to live with you', it doesn't bode well for living together.

In any event, a trial period is a good idea – call it a holiday. If you do go down this route, your home may need some adaptations: see the section on adaptations on pages 116–122.

Another possibility, if finances permit, is to build an annexe to your home for the person with arthritis to move into. This can provide the ideal compromise, giving you both independence while maintaining close contact.

Care homes

People often regard 'going into a home' as a last resort, and may be sceptical about the quality and value of the care provided. Nevertheless, there are homes that provide good care, and one of those might be the best option. Independence is lost but, in a good home, probably not to the degree that might be feared. Carers are strangers – which some people regard as an advantage – and they ought to be professionals.

If this is the option the person with arthritis prefers, the best thing you can do as a carer is to ensure that the home and its facilities are thoroughly checked out. There are care homes run by the private sector, by voluntary organisations and by the local authority. Many homes in the voluntary sector are for particular groups of people – war veterans, for example; one of these may be appropriate.

The best way to find a home is probably by word of mouth but social workers, the local 'Patient Advice and Liaison Service' (PALS) and local voluntary organisations can also help. You should also contact the local regional office of the National Care Standards Commission (NCSC). The NCSC (national address on page 147) is responsible for inspecting care homes. (In 2004 it will amalgamate with the Social Services Inspectorate to become the Commission for Social Care Inspection.) You can ask the local office for a list of care homes in the area and also for the inspection reports of the homes in which you are interested.

It is vital to visit the homes being considered. Some will prefer you to make an appointment but others will suggest that you call in any time. It may be possible for the person with arthritis to arrange to stay for a short 'holiday', to get a better feel of the home before making a final decision.

Issues to consider

- The 'ethos' of the home – do they encourage residents to make their own decisions? Can they, for example, eat what they want? Is there a residents' committee?
- Privacy – private phones? Single or shared rooms? What about personal possessions?
- Flexibility – how fixed are visiting times, bedtimes, mealtimes and so on?
- Facilities – for example, are there outings and recreational opportunities, communal living rooms, books, newspapers, mobile library?
- Cost – the contract between the home and the resident should state clearly the fees and what extras might apply.
- Environment – the considerations of access to local shops and transport and so on, discussed under retirement housing (pages 126–127), apply here too.

For more *i*nformation

 Age Concern Factsheet 29 *Finding Care Home Accommodation* (see page 157 for details of how to obtain factsheets).

 Relatives and Residents Association checklist *Questions to Ask* (see address on page 149).

Paying for care in a care home

Care arranged by the NHS

If the NHS arranges care for your relative in a home which provides nursing care, they will be regarded as a long-stay NHS patient and the NHS will pay in full for the care. In England and Wales the NHS funds the care provided by a registered nurse in a care home providing nursing. In England there are three bands (£40, £75 or £120 a week in 2003), depending on the level of nursing your relative is assessed as needing. In Wales there is one level (£100 in 2003). In Scotland local authorities meet nursing and personal care costs (see below).

Care arranged by the local authority

Before the local authority can offer any financial help your relative will need to have an assessment of their needs (see pages 86–90). If the local authority agrees to arrange a place for your relative in a private or voluntary care home, it will be responsible for paying the full fee to the home and assessing your relative's income and savings to see how much they must pay towards the fees. If your relative has savings of more than an upper capital limit (£19,500 in England in 2003) they will have to pay the full fee until their savings reach that amount.

In Scotland for people aged 65 or over the full fee is the living and accommodation costs only as the local authority meets the personal care (£145 per week in 2003) and nursing costs (£65 in 2003) of the home. For people under 65 it just meets the nursing costs.

If your relative has £16,000 or less and is under 60, they may be able to receive Income Support as well as financial support from the local authority towards the fees. If your relative is 60 or over, they may be able to get Pension Credit even if their capital is above that amount.

If your relative owns their own home, the value will normally be taken into account unless the house has certain other occupants, including their partner or a 'relative' who is either disabled or aged 60 or over. The local authority can also take account of certain assets which your relative might have transferred to someone else in order to pay less for their care.

When one of a couple enters a care home, the local authority will assess the amount the resident has to pay solely on the resident's income and savings. However, a spouse (but not an unmarried partner) is a 'liable relative' and so may have to contribute towards the cost of care. There are, however, no national rules about how much a spouse must pay; the local authority will try to reach a 'voluntary agreement'. If your relative has an occupational or personal pension and their spouse is not living in the care home with them, the local authority will ignore half the pension when assessing your relative's income.

Paying for care privately

Even someone who can arrange and pay for a care home themselves is advised not to move into one until they have asked social services for an assessment. A care home may not be the best option. Social services may be able suggest ways that would allow continued independent living. They will also be happy to provide information about homes to people arranging their own care.

Anyone making their own arrangements should also think about what might happen as their money runs out. It may be possible to stay in the home chosen but, if social services consider that it is not suitable or it costs too much, they may arrange a place elsewhere. If it is likely that capital will fall below the capital limit, it is sensible to talk to the social services department before moving into a home.

For more *i*nformation

i Age Concern Factsheets (see page 157 for details of how to obtain factsheets):

10 *Local Authority Charging Procedures for Care Homes*

20 *Continuing NHS Health Care, 'Free' Nursing Care and Intermediate Care*

38 *Treatment of the Former Home as Capital for People in Care Homes*

39 *Paying for Care in a Care Home if You Have a Partner*

40 *Transfer of Assets and Paying for Care in a Care Home.*

Getting about

By car

Many people with arthritis can drive. Often, all that is needed are a few features that are now standard on many cars – power steering and automatic transmission, for example. There is also an abundance of adaptations and aids available, which means that even the most specialist needs can be met.

When buying or leasing a car, it is vital to try it out thoroughly, having made sure that it meets all needs. Consider, for example, whether the car should have two or four doors: in a two-door car, the seat can be slid further back and the door is usually bigger and opens wider; but this will make the door heavier and perhaps more difficult to shut. Look out also for the door sills: high sills can make it harder to get in and out of the car. And how easy will it be to load and unload a wheelchair?

A very good way to find out what one's needs are is to get an assessment from an approved mobility centre. For more information about cars and assessments, contact the Mobility Advice and Vehicle Information Service (MAVIS) at the address on page 147.

People receiving the higher rate of the mobility component of Disability Living Allowance (see pages 108–109) can generally use it to buy or lease a car from Motability (see address on page 147), the government initiative to get disabled people mobile.

Concessions that may be available to disabled motorists include:

- exemption from VAT on necessary adaptations to a car;
- exemption from car tax (Vehicle Excise Duty) – the Disability Living Allowance Unit will automatically send your relative an application form (DLA 403) for a VED exemption certificate if they receive the higher rate of the mobility component of DLA;
- the use of disabled parking bays; and
- the Blue Badge scheme (previously known as the Orange Badge scheme) which provides a national system of parking concessions; applications are made to the local authority social services department.

By public transport

Trains

Facilities on trains vary widely. Newer trains are designed to allow full access for people with disabilities, including people in wheelchairs. However, older trains may be less accessible and people in wheelchairs may, in some cases, have to travel in the guard's van. Some InterCity routes now have wheelchair accessible on-train toilets but toilets on older trains and local services are not accessible at present. Many mainline stations are accessible but facilities and availability of staff also vary widely. Some smaller stations are unstaffed and assistance cannot be provided.

There is a code of practice which is intended to offer people with disabilities a universal common standard of service. It applies to people who have advised in advance of their travel arrangements (at least 24 hours notice is usually required). To find out which train company to contact, telephone National Rail Enquiries on 0845 748 4950.

A free leaflet called *Rail Travel for Disabled Passengers* is available from main stations and travel agents (or from the Disabled Persons Railcard Office at the address on page 145).

Buses and coaches

All new buses have to be accessible. However, it will be some years before all vehicles in service will comply. Contact the local bus company for details of accessible buses. Some cities have Mobility Buses, which are accessible to people in wheelchairs.

All new large coaches will have to be wheelchair accessible from January 2005, but, again, it will be many years before they all are. Existing coaches cannot usually carry wheelchair passengers unless the coach has been specially adapted. Many operators will provide assistance for disabled people but you usually have to give seven days notice.

By air

Airlines are also becoming more aware of the needs of disabled people. The key point here, as with all public transport, is to be very specific in advance about what is needed and when. For example, what arrangements need to be made for a wheelchair? Your travel agent should be able to tell you what facilities are available. It is probably worth double-checking with the airline and/or the airport nearer the departure time to make sure that the relevant people have been informed (or have not forgotten) about any requirements.

There is a website with information on the services offered to people with disabilities by 50 airlines. It is at www.everybody.co.uk

By sea

As with other forms of transport, facilities for people with disabilities when travelling by ship can vary widely, both at terminals and on board. Check with the travel agent and/or the shipping company to find out what facilities are available and to let them know of any requirements for you or the person you are caring for.

It is irritating that few transport operators seem able to offer the sort of blanket access that would enable disabled people to use their facilities on the same basis as non-disabled people. However, with advance warning their 'customer care' strategies come into play and most will try to be helpful.

Schemes to help with transport

If your relative cannot use ordinary public transport, there a number of door-to-door transport schemes that they may be able to use for local journeys:

- Dial-a-ride schemes enable disabled people to book lifts in a minibus or similar vehicle and are available in many areas. The local disability advice organisation should be able to provide more information.

- Social car schemes use volunteers driving their own cars to take people to visit the doctor or to go shopping, for example. They are often run by the local Council for Voluntary Service or volunteer bureau but your relative will need a letter from their GP or social services to say that they cannot use public transport.

- Shopmobility schemes are available in many town centres. They will lend a wheelchair/scooter to anyone with a mobility problem. The user can often park free or be met at the bus station or taxi rank by prior arrangement.

- Taxicard schemes are available to disabled people living in most London boroughs who are unable to use public transport – contact the local authority to see if it runs such a scheme.

Tripscope (address on page 150) is a charity which specialises in giving information and advice on travel and transport for older and disabled people. It is not a travel or booking agency but can help you plan a journey so that it will be as easy as possible.

For more *i*nformation

 Age Concern Factsheet 26 *Travel Information for Older People* (see page 157 for details of how to obtain factsheets).

 Contact **Tripscope** at the address on page 150.

 For information about local schemes to help with transport, contact the local council or the **Community Transport Association** at the address on page 143.

Taking a break

Taking a break – or respite care – is often cited by carers as the single most important thing in making their job possible. Tony has been married for 56 years to Sheila and now cares for her. He thinks a little time apart is invaluable.

Tony

'We have a Crossroads carer once a week and a daily paid carer, which takes a lot of the weight off my shoulders. It gives us both our own time. I like to paint, read or do crosswords. It's imperative to have a break, even from the person you love most in the world.'

Tom and teenager Jenny agree.

Tom

'The toughest thing about caring is not getting a break. I don't mind taking care of everything on a day-to-day basis – that keeps me busy – but it's the fact that it never stops. As you get older you have less energy and get tired. We haven't had a holiday since I retired. I think I'm pretty resourceful and our generation are good at making do but even so ...'

Jenny

'I'm involved with the Edinburgh Young Carers group so I can chat and go out with other people in the same position. That helps a lot. But a befriender to take my mum out too would really make a difference.'

Everybody needs some time off occasionally – and if you're a carer you need it more than most. But according to figures quoted by Crossroads, 33 per cent of carers say that they have not had a break in the last two years. And some carers even feel guilty for wanting a break.

If you feel like this, let your guilt go and examine the situation objectively. Without a break, any human being will become tired. If you are tired, you can make mistakes or become ill – two things that are no good at all for you or the person you are caring for. If that doesn't convince you, what about the benefits to the other person? They could do with a break from you too. A change of scene, some time with other people, and you'll both feel better afterwards.

The options for breaks include care at home, day care away from home, residential breaks and holidays.

Care at home

You have the right to have your own needs assessed (see page 74) and one of these could well be the need for a break. This may take the form of services or direct payments with which to purchase care. The *Carers and Disabled Children Act 2000* introduced vouchers which are given to the cared-for person to enable them to purchase assistance when their carer takes a break – these are intended to create a situation where the carer can have control of when they take a break and the cared-for person can have control of what help they get. Social services may offer a home help or home care assistant, meals-on-wheels or a sitter or care attendant. If necessary, point out to them the advantages to their budget of supporting you as a carer now, rather than meeting the full care costs of the person you care for in the future because you cannot cope. GPs may be able to arrange some care at home, such as visits from the community nurse to help with nursing care.

If another member of your family or a friend cannot stand in for you, explore local sitting services. Many social services, health trusts and voluntary organisations can provide sitters, offering helpers for a few hours a week. They can just sit with the person or they may provide help with getting up or preparing meals. Most are experienced although untrained. There may be a charge. For more care, consider a local authority care attendant. Again, there may be a charge.

There may be a care attendant scheme in your area, run by Crossroads – Caring for the Carers (see national address on page 144) and the Leonard Cheshire Foundation also has a Care At Home service (see national address on page 147).

Day care away from home

This can be a regular daily or weekly break or a week every few months. It may be provided by voluntary organisations or by the health service or local authority. There might be a charge. Day care can be at a day centre or a lunch and social club, or at a day hospital if specialist medical treatment or care is needed. Transport may be provided, for which there may be a charge.

Residential breaks

To get a good break for a few days, there is the possibility of temporary residential care for the person for whom you care. It will give you both a change, and give you the house to yourself for a while if you live together.

It may involve a short stay in a hospital, a hospice or a care home. Respite stays in NHS hospitals or a hospice run by a charity are usually free. If the local authority arranges a stay in a care home, there will usually be a flat-rate nightly fee. For a stay over eight weeks, there will normally be a means test.

There are a few schemes enabling the person you care for to stay with another family. These are mainly for children but there are some for adults. Ask social services about family-based respite care whereby people go and stay with another carefully selected and trained family.

Holidays

You can go on holiday either together or separately. There is a little financial help available from social services, although eligibility criteria can be strict and some authorities do not make grants at all. There are home exchange schemes and some holiday companies that specialise in singles or in special needs. These are listed in the Carers UK leaflet *Taking a Break*.

RADAR (address on page 149) publishes several holiday guides, giving information on places to stay in the UK (including information on the availability of ground-floor bedrooms, lifts, size of entrance doors), holidays in the rest of Europe, access to air travel, ferries, rail and coach travel and insurance.

Arthritis Care runs four hotels in the UK. They are fully accessible and aim to offer stress-free holidays in beautiful coastal settings. You don't need to be a member of the charity to book.

A number of Age Concerns locally run their own holidays, often aimed at more active older people but which may also be suitable for those who have a disability.

The Holiday Care Service (address on page 146) is a charity which provides specialist information on holidays for disabled people and their carers. It publishes a variety of information sheets on topics such as how to find voluntary or paid helpers/carers for holidays and travel. It also has a reservations service for accessible hotels in the UK.

Organising a break can be expensive, which is another good reason to make sure you are claiming all the benefits you are both entitled to. Charities may be able to help too – look at the Holiday Care Service information sheet which details national charities which have been known to give grants towards holidays or contact the Association of Charity Officers or Charity Search (at the addresses on page 141 and 143).

For further *i*nformation

ⓘ Contact the **Holiday Care Service** (address on page 146).

ⓘ Carers UK leaflet *Taking a Break* (address on page 143).

ⓘ *Arthritis Care Hotels: Easy Breaks* is available from the address on page 141.

7 Five things for every carer

Hopefully this book hasn't put you off becoming a carer but, rather, has helped you appreciate exactly what is being taken on and suggested ways to help you cope with the challenges. Probably the five most useful things a carer can do are summarised here.

■ Get a carer's assessment from the local social services department. They can assess the type of support you need, such as meals-on-wheels, respite care and practical help in the home. This assessment is your right.

■ Find out about – and use – respite care.

■ Make sure that your doctor, social services, pharmacist and employer know your situation.

■ Talk about how you feel with someone in the family who understands the situation or with a close friend, GP or counsellor. Try the Arthritis Care Freephone Helpline on 0808 800 4050 (12pm–4pm, Monday to Friday) or the Carers UK CarersLine on 0808 808 7777 (10am–12 noon & 2pm–4pm, Monday to Friday).

■ Check out what Carers UK can offer. You should certainly make sure that you join some sort of an organisation or group where you can meet other carers, while encouraging the person you are caring for to join a group such as Arthritis Care where they can meet other people with arthritis.

Useful addresses

Abbeyfield Society
*Housing association
specialising in bedsitters/flats
for older people in shared
houses, with warden and
housekeeper available.*

53 Victoria Street
St Albans
Herts AL1 3UW
Tel: 01727 857536
Website:
www.abbeyfield.com

Arthritis Care
*Provides information, support,
training, fun and social
contact. The first port of call
for anyone with arthritis.
There are many smaller
organisations for particular
types of arthritis – Arthritis
Care's Helpline can provide
details.*

18 Stephenson Way
London NW1 2HD
Tel: 020 7380 6500
(switchboard)
Publications (including
Arthritis News):
020 7380 6540
Freephone Helpline
0808 800 4050 (12pm–4pm,
Monday to Friday)
24-hour Info Line:
0845 600 6868
Website: www.arthritiscare.org.uk

Arthritis Research Campaign
*The leading arthritis research
organisation in the UK, funding
much research and also
producing useful information
for patients.*

Copeman House
St Mary's Court
St Mary's Gate
Chesterfield S41 7TD
Tel: 0870 850 5000
Website: www.arc.org.uk

Association of Charity Officers
*Provides information about
charities that make grants to
individuals in need.*

Unicorn House
Station Close
Potters Bar
Hertfordshire EN6 3JW
Tel: 01707 651777
Website: www.aco.uk.net

141

Association of Reflexologists
*The largest independent
organisation of reflexologists.*

27 Old Gloucester Street
London WC1N 3XX
Tel: 0870 567 3320
Website: www.aor.org.uk

**Association of Traditional
Chinese Medicine**
*Many Chinese-trained practitioners
of herbal medicine are members.*

78 Haverstock Hill
London NW3 2BE
Tel: 020 7284 2898

**Benefit Enquiry Line for people
with disabilities**
*State benefits information line
for ill or disabled people and
their carers.*

Freephone: 0800 88 22 00
(8.30am–6.30pm, Monday to
Friday)

British Acupuncture Council
*Regulatory body of
acupuncturists.*

63 Jeddo Road
London W12 9HQ
Tel: 020 8735 0400
Website:
www.acupuncture.org.uk

**British Association for
Counselling and Psychotherapy**
*For a list of counsellors
and organisations in
your area.*

1 Regent Place
Rugby
Warwickshire CV21 2PJ
Tel: 0870 443 5252
Website: www.bacp.co.uk

British Chiropractic Association
Regulatory body of chiropractors.

Blagrave House
17 Blagrave Street
Reading RG1 1QB
Tel: 0118 950 5950
Website:
www.chiropractic-uk.co.uk

**British Homeopathic Association
(incorporating the Homeopathic
Trust)**
*For names of homeopathic
practitioners.*

15 Clerkenwell Close
London EC1R 0AA
Tel: 020 7566 7800
Website:
www.trusthomeopathy.org

British Society for Rheumatology
The UK professional organisation
for people working in
rheumatology and related fields.

41 Eagle Street
London WC1R 4TL
Tel: 020 7242 3313
Website:
www.rheumatology.org.uk

Carers UK
Provides a wide range of
information and support to all
carers. Can put you in touch
with other carers and carers'
groups in your area.

20–25 Glasshouse Yard
London EC1A 4JT
Tel: 020 7490 8818 (admin)
CarersLine: 0808 808 7777
(10am–12 noon & 2pm–4pm,
Monday to Friday)
Website:
www.carersonline.org.uk

Centre for Accessible
Environments
Gives advice on accessible
design for buildings.

60 Gainsford Street
London SE1 2NY
Tel: 020 7357 8182
Website: www.cae.org.uk

Charity Search
Helps link older people with
charities that may provide
grants to individuals.
Applications in writing are
preferred.

25 Portview Road
Avonmouth
Bristol BS11 9LD
Tel: 0117 982 4060
(9am–3pm, Monday to
Thursday)

Chartered Society of Physiotherapy
For chartered physiotherapists
in your area.

14 Bedford Row
London WC1R 4ED
Tel: 020 7306 6666
Website:
www.csp.org.uk

Community Transport Association
For information about local
schemes to help with transport.

Highbank
Halton Street
Hyde
Cheshire SK14 2NY
Tel: 0161 351 1475
Advice: 0161 367 8780
Website:
www.communitytransport.com

143

Counsel and Care
*Advice on remaining at home
or about care homes.*

Twyman House
16 Bonny Street
London NW1 9PG
Tel: 020 7241 8555 (admin)
Advice Line: 0845 300 7585
(10am–12.30pm & 2pm–4pm,
Monday to Friday)
Website:
www.counselandcare.org.uk

**Crossroads – Caring for the
Carers**
*Has nearly 200 schemes across
England and Wales providing
practical support to carers in
the home.*

10 Regent Place
Rugby
Warwickshire CV21 2PN
Tel: 01788 573653
Website: www.crossroads.org.uk

Disability Alliance
Information on welfare benefits.

Universal House
88–94 Wentworth Street
London E1 7SA
Tel: 020 7247 8776 (10am–4pm,
Monday to Friday)
Rights advice line:
020 7247 8763 (2pm–4pm,
Monday and Wednesday)
Website:
www.disabilityalliance.org

**Disablement Information and
Advice Lines (DIAL UK)**
*For your nearest local group,
giving information and advice
about disability.*

St Catherine's Hospital
Tickhill Road
Doncaster
South Yorkshire DN4 8QN
Tel: 01302 310123
Website: www.dialuk.org.uk

Disability Sport England
*National agency that
encourages sport from
local to national level.*

N17 Studio
Unit 4G
784–788 High Road
London N17 0DA
Tel: 020 8801 4466
Website:
www.disabilitysport.org.uk

Disability Wales
National association of disability groups working to promote the rights, recognition and support of all disabled people in Wales.

Wernddu Court
Caerphilly Business Park
Van Road
Caerphilly CF83 3ED
Tel: 029 2088 7325
Website: www.dwac.demon.co.uk

Disabled Living Centres Council
For a centre near you, where you can see aids and equipment.

Redbank House
4 St Chad's Street
Manchester M8 8QA
Tel: 0161 834 1044
Website: www.dlcc.org.uk

Disabled Living Foundation
Information and advice about aids to help people cope with a disability.

380–384 Harrow Road
London W9 2HU
Tel: 020 7289 6111
Helpline: 0845 130 9177
(10am–4pm, Monday to Friday)
Website: www.dlf.org.uk

Disabled Persons Railcard Office
For a railcard offering concessionary fares. An application form and booklet Rail Travel for Disabled Passengers *can be found at main stations or from this address.*

PO Box 1YT
Newcastle upon Tyne NE99 1YT
Helpline: 0191 269 0303
Website: www.disabledpersons
-railcard.co.uk

Elderly Accommodation Counsel
National charity offering computerised information about all forms of accommodation for older people.

3rd Floor
89 Albert Embankment
London SE1 7TP
Helpline: 020 7820 1343
Website: www.housingcare.org

Energy Action Grants Agency (EAGA)
Administers the Warm Front Grants in England, the Home Energy Efficiency Scheme in Wales and the Warm Deal and Central Heating Programme in Scotland.

Freepost NEA 12054
Newcastle upon Tyne NE1 7HA
Freephone: 0800 316 6011
(England)
0800 316 2815 (Wales)
0800 072 0150 (Scotland)
Website: www.eaga.co.uk

English Heritage
For a guide for people with
disabilities.

Customer Services Department
PO Box 569
Swindon SN2 2YP
Tel: 0870 333 1181
Website:
www.english-heritage.org.uk

foundations
The national co-ordinating body
for home improvement agencies.

Bleaklow House
Howard Town Mill
Glossop SK13 8HT
Tel: 01457 891909
Website: www.foundations.uk.com

General Chiropractic Council
The statutory body regulating
practitioners of chiropractic.

344–354 Gray's Inn Road
London WC1X 8BP
Tel: 020 7713 5155
Website: www.gcc-uk.org

General Osteopathic Council
For advice on finding a
registered osteopath.

Osteopathic House
176 Tower Bridge Road
London SE1 3LU
Tel: 020 7357 6655
Website: www.osteopathy.org.uk

Holiday Care Service
Information and advice about
holidays for older or disabled
people and their carers. Has a
database of respite care facilities
in the UK.

7th Floor, Sunley House
4 Bedford Park
Croydon CR0 2AP
Tel: 0845 124 9971
Website: www.holidaycare.org.uk

Independent Living (1993) Fund
May provide top-up funding to
severely disabled people.
Applications must be made before
the age of 66.

PO Box 183
Nottingham NG8 3RD
Tel: 0115 942 8191

Institute for Complementary
Medicine
Information and advice about
complementary therapy. Please
send an sae and state the
therapy you are interested in.

PO Box 194
London SE16 1QZ
Tel: 020 7237 5165
(10am–3pm, Monday to Friday)
Website: www.icmedicine.co.uk

Leonard Cheshire Foundation
Charity providing services for
disabled people in the UK.

30 Millbank
London SW1P 4QD
Tel: 020 7802 8200
Website:
www.leonard-cheshire.org.uk

Lupus UK
UK-wide charity that supports
people with lupus.

St James House
Eastern Road
Romford
Essex RM1 3NH
Tel: 01708 731251
Website: www.lupusuk.com

**MAVIS (Mobility Advice and
Vehicle Information Service)**
Driving assessments and advice.

Department for Transport
MacAdam Avenue
Old Wokingham Road
Crowthorne
Berkshire RG45 6XD
Tel: 01344 661000
Website: www.mobility-
unit.dft.gov.uk

Motability
Advice and help about cars,
scooters and wheelchairs for
disabled people.

Goodman House
Station Approach
Harlow
Essex CM20 2ET
Tel: 01279 635666
Website: www.motability.co.uk

**National Care Standards
Commission (NCSC)**
Responsible for inspecting and
registering care homes. Contact
the head office for details of your
local office.

St Nicholas Buildings
St Nicholas Street
Newcastle upon Tyne NE1 1NB
Helpline: 0191 233 3556
(8am–6pm, Monday to Friday)
Website:
www.carestandards.org.uk

**National Centre for Independent
Living**
Provides advice on independent
living and direct payments, and
details of your local Centre for
Independent Living

250 Kennington Lane
London SE11 5RD
Tel: 020 7587 1663
Website: www.ncil.org.uk

147

NHS Direct
*First point of contact to find out
about NHS services.*

Tel: 0845 46 47
Website: www.nhsdirect.nhs.uk

**National Institute of Medical
Herbalists**
*To find a practitioner of Western
herbal medicine.*

56 Longbrook Street
Exeter
Devon EX4 6AH
Tel: 01392 426022
Website: www.nimh.org.uk

National Osteoporosis Society
*For information about osteoporosis
and a list of specialist centres.*

Camerton
Bath BA2 0PJ
Helpline: 0845 450 0230
Website: www.nos.org.uk

National Trust
*Contact the Disability Officer
for information.*

36 Queen Anne's Gate
London SW1H 9AS
Tel: 020 7447 6742/3
Website:
www.nationaltrust.org.uk

**Pensions Advisory Service
(OPAS)**
*A voluntary organisation which
gives advice and information about
occupational and personal pensions
and helps sort out problems.*

11 Belgrave Road
London SW1V 1RB
Tel: 0845 601 2923
Website: www.opas.org.uk

Princess Royal Trust for Carers
*Aims to make it easier for carers
to cope by providing information,
support and practical help. Your
phone book may list a local branch.*

142 Minories
London EC3N 1LB
Tel: 020 7480 7788
Website: www.carers.org

Psoriatic Arthropathy Alliance
*Helps people with psoriatic
arthritis, and raises awareness
of the condition.*

PO Box 111
St Albans
Herts AL2 3JQ
Tel: 0870 770 3212
Website: www.paalliance.org

RADAR (Royal Association for Disability and Rehabilitation)
Campaigning and advisory disability body. Information and publications on topics such as aids and mobility, holidays and leisure.

12 City Forum
250 City Road
London EC1V 8AF
Tel: 020 7250 3222
Website: www.radar.org.uk

Relatives and Residents Association
Advice and support for relatives of people in a care home or in hospital long term.

24 The Ivories
6–18 Northampton Street
Islington
London N1 2HY
Helpline: 020 7359 8136

REMAP
For customised aids and gadgets.

National Organiser
Hazeldene
Ightham
Sevenoaks
Kent TN15 9AD
Tel: 0845 1300 456
Website: www.remap.org.uk

RoSPA (Royal Society for the Prevention of Accidents)
Advice and publications on preventing accidents.

Edgbaston Park
353 Bristol Road
Edgbaston
Birmingham B5 7ST
Tel: 0121 248 2000
Website: www.rospa.com

Society of Homeopaths
For a list of homeopathic practitioners.

4A Artizan Road
Northampton NN1 4HU
Tel: 01604 621400
Website:
www.homeopathy-soh.org

Sport England
For addresses and information about all sport.

16 Upper Woburn Place
London WC1H 0QP
Tel: 020 7273 1500
Website: www.sportengland.org

Thrive
Advice, information and training on gardening for people with disabilities or special needs.

Geoffrey Udall Centre
Beech Hill
Reading RG7 2AT
Tel: 0118 988 5688
Website: www.thrive.org.uk

Tripscope
A travel information service for older and disabled people.

The Vassall Centre
Gill Avenue
Bristol BS16 2QQ
Helpline: 08457 585641
Website: www.tripscope.org.uk

UK Home Care Association (UKHCA)
For information about member organisations providing home care.

42b Banstead Road
Carshalton Beeches
Surrey SM5 3NW
Tel: 020 8288 1551
Website: www.ukhca.co.uk

West of England Centre for Inclusive Living
Advice and a guide for users of the direct payments scheme.

Leinster Avenue
Knowle West
Bristol BS4 1AR
Tel: 0117 903 8900

150

About Age Concern

This book is one of a wide range of publications produced by Age Concern England, the National Council on Ageing. Age Concern works on behalf of all older people and believes later life should be fulfilling and enjoyable. For too many this is impossible. As the leading charitable movement in the UK concerned with ageing and older people, Age Concern finds effective ways to change that situation.

Where possible, we enable older people to solve problems themselves, providing as much or as little support as they need. A network of local Age Concerns, supported by many thousands of volunteers, provides community-based services such as lunch clubs, day centres and home visiting.

Nationally, we take a lead role in campaigning, parliamentary work, policy analysis, research, specialist information and advice provision, and publishing. Innovative programmes promote healthier lifestyles and provide older people with opportunities to give the experience of a lifetime back to their communities.

Age Concern is dependent on donations, covenants and legacies.

Age Concern England
1268 London Road
London SW16 4ER
Tel: 020 8765 7200
Fax: 020 8765 7211
Website:
www.ageconcern.org.uk

Age Concern Scotland
113 Rose Street
Edinburgh EH2 3DT
Tel: 0131 220 3345
Fax: 0131 220 2779
Website:
www.ageconcernscotland.org.uk

Age Concern Cymru
4th Floor
1 Cathedral Road
Cardiff CF11 9SD
Tel: 029 2037 1566
Fax: 029 2039 9562
Website:
www.accymru.org.uk

Age Concern Northern Ireland
3 Lower Crescent
Belfast BT7 1NR
Tel: 028 9024 5729
Fax: 028 9023 5497
Website:
www.ageconcernni.org

About Arthritis Care

Arthritis Care is the largest UK-wide voluntary organisation working with and for people with arthritis. In fact, people with arthritis are involved at every level. Arthritis Care is committed to improving the lives of all people with arthritis through representation, information and support, training and inclusion.

Our vision is clear. We are working hard to ensure the nine million people with arthritis in the UK are included in society and given access to the same opportunities as everyone else. We are striving to create an environment which enables people with arthritis to manage their condition by providing them with accurate and appropriate information, support through our network of branches and our helpline, and self-management skills through our training service.

Arthritis Care:

- provides a helpline service by telephone, letter and email, weekdays 12pm–4pm on a Freephone helpline (0808 800 4050). It is also available 10am–4pm charged at the national rate. Tel: 020 7380 6555. Email: Helplines@arthritiscare.org.uk;
- offers a range of self-management and personal development training courses for people with arthritis of all ages to enable people to be in control of their arthritis;
- produces a range of helpful publications including the bi-monthly magazine, *Arthritis News*, and a website;
- campaigns for greater awareness of the needs of all people with arthritis;
- has over 500 branches and groups; and
- runs four accessible hotels in the UK.

For further information about Arthritis Care, call our 24-hour information line on 0845 600 6868 or log onto our website at www.arthritiscare.org.uk

Arthritis Care, 18 Stephenson Way, London NW1 2HD. Reg Charity No 206563.

Other books in this series

The Carer's Handbook: What to do and who to turn to
Marina Lewycka
£6.99 0-86242-366-X

Choices for the carer of an elderly relative
Marina Lewycka
£6.99 0-86242-375-9

Caring for someone with depression
Toni Battison
£6.99 0-86242-389-9

Caring for someone with cancer
Toni Battison
£6.99 0-86242-382-1

Caring for someone with a sight problem
Marina Lewycka
£6.99 0-86242-381-3

Caring for someone with a hearing loss
Marina Lewycka
£6.99 0-86242-380-5

Caring for someone who is dying
Penny Mares
£6.99 0-86242-370-8

Caring for someone with a heart problem
Toni Battison
£6.99 0-86242-371-6

Caring for someone with diabetes
Marina Lewycka
£6.99 0-86242-374-0

Caring for someone at a distance
Julie Spencer-Cingöz
£6.99 0-86242-367-8

Caring for someone who has had a stroke
Philip Coyne with Penny Mares
£6.99 0-86242-369-4

Caring for someone with an alcohol problem
Mike Ward
£6.99 0-86242-372-4

Caring for someone with dementia
Jane Brotchie
£6.99 0-86242-368-6

Caring for someone with memory loss
Toni Battison
£6.99 0-86242-358-9

Publications from Age Concern Books

Know Your Complementary Therapies
Eileen Inge Herzberg

Written in clear, jargon-free language, this book provides an introduction to complementary therapies, including acupuncture, herbal medicine, aromatherapy, spiritual healing, homeopathy and osteopathy. Uniquely focusing on complementary therapies and older people, the book helps readers to decide which therapies are best suited to their needs, and where to go for help.

£9.99 0-86242-309-0

Staying Sane: Managing the Stress of Caring
Tanya Arroba and Lesley Bell

The aim of this book is to increase the positive rewards associated with caring and demystify the topic of stress. Complete with case studies and checklists, the book helps carers to develop a clear strategy towards dealing positively with stress.

£14.99 0-86242-267-1

Alive and Kicking: The Carer's Guide to Exercises for Older People
Julie Sobczak with Susie Dinan and Piers Simey

Regular activity is essential in helping older people to remain agile and independent. This illustrated book contains a wealth of ideas on topics such as motivating the exerciser, safety issues and medical advice, exercise warm-ups and injury prevention and head to toe chair exercises. The book also provides handy tips and ideas on stretching and relaxation techniques, using props and how to make exercise fun.

£11.99 0-86242-289-2

Your Rights: A Guide to Money Benefits for Older People
Sally West

A highly acclaimed annual guide to the State benefits available to older people. Contains current information on State Pensions, means-tested benefits and disability benefits, among other matters, and provides advice on how to claim.

For further information please telephone 0870 44 22 120.

If you would like to order any of these titles, please write to the address below, enclosing a cheque or money order for the appropriate amount (plus £1.95 p&p) made payable to Age Concern England. Credit card orders may be made on 0870 44 22 120. Books can also be ordered online at www.ageconcern.org.uk/shop

Age Concern Books
Units 5 and 6
Industrial Estate
Brecon
Powys LD3 8LA

Customised editions

Age Concern Books is pleased to offer a free 'customisation' service for anyone wishing to purchase 500 or more copies of the title. This gives you the option to have a unique front cover design featuring your organisation's logo and corporate colours, or adding your logo to the current cover design. You can also insert an additional four pages of text for a small additional fee. Existing clients include many of the biggest names in British industry, retailing and finance, the trades unions, educational establishments, the statutory and voluntary sectors, and welfare associations.

For full details, please contact Sue Henning, Age Concern Books, Astral House, 1268 London Road, London SW16 4ER. Fax: 020 8765 7211. Email: hennings@ace.org.uk

Visit our website at www.ageconcern.org.uk/shop

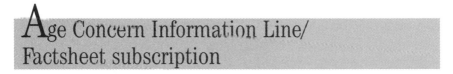

Age Concern Information Line/ Factsheet subscription

Age Concern produces more than 45 comprehensive factsheets designed to answer many of the questions older people (or those advising them) may have. These include money and benefits, health, community care, leisure and education, and housing. For up to five free factsheets, telephone: 0800 00 99 66 (7am–7pm, seven days a week, every day of the year). Alternatively you may prefer to write to Age Concern, FREEPOST (SWB 30375), ASHBURTON, Devon TQ13 7ZZ.

For professionals working with older people, the factsheets are available on an annual subscription service, which includes updates throughout the year. For further details and costs of the subscription, please contact Age Concern at the above address.

Bulk order discounts

Age Concern Books is pleased to offer a discount on orders totalling 50 or more copies of the same title. For details, please contact Age Concern Books on Tel: 0870 44 22 120.

We hope that this publication has been useful to you. If so, we would very much like to hear from you. Alternatively, if you feel that we could add or change anything, then please write and tell us, using the following Freepost address: Age Concern, FREEPOST CN1794, London SW16 4BR.

Index